THE GREEN KITCHEN HANDBOOK

*Practical Advice, References, and Sources for
Transforming the Center of Your Home
into a Healthful, Livable Place*

Foreword by Meryl Streep

*Annie Berthold-Bond
and Mothers & Others for a Livable Planet*

HarperPerennial
A Division of HarperCollinsPublishers

HarperCollins books may be purchased for educational, business, or sales promotional use. For information please write: Special Markets Department, HarperCollins Publishers, Inc., 10 East 53rd Street, New York, NY 10022.

FIRST EDITION

Designed by Toshiko S. Furuta

Library of Congress Cataloging-in-Publication Data

Berthold-Bond, Annie.
   The green kitchen handbook : practical advice, references, and sources for transforming the center of your home into a healthful, livable place / Anne Berthold-Bond and Mothers & Others for a Livable Planet. — 1st ed.
      p.   cm.
   Includes index.
   ISBN 0-06-095186-9
   1. Nutrition.   2. Green products.   3. Kitchens.   I. Mothers & Others for a Livable Planet, Inc.   II. Title.
   TX353.B494   1997   96-43028
   613.2—dc20

97 98 99 00 01 ❖/RRD 10 9 8 7 6 5 4 3 2 1

*This book is dedicated
to all who buy and eat food
from sustainable farms and gardens*

Contents

5 Preserving the Foods of the Harvest *180*

Foreword

The kitchen is the center of our family's home, the place where everyone—kids, parents, and friends—comes to replenish and refuel, to laugh and tell stories, to argue and cry, and most of all to settle and repose. Our kitchen tells its own very special story, about our family, its values, the way it works and thinks. How we treat our homes—what we bring into them and how we care for them—affects how we feel about ourselves and others.

My kitchen has changed over the last few years, since my involvement with Mothers & Others for a Livable Planet. I pay much more attention to where and how the food I buy for my family is grown. I try to buy locally grown, organic, and whole foods. When I can, I make meals from scratch, so I have learned to stock my pantry with the basics.

As my family's food-buying habits have changed, so has our diet. We eat less meat and do not miss it; we have discovered many delicious, equally nutritious alternatives. *The Green Kitchen Handbook* describes each of them, in scrumptious detail, including how to shop for, store, and prepare them.

The book also may open your eyes, as it did mine, to the range of natural whole sweeteners that are far better for you but just as tasty as the refined white sugar with which most of us are familiar. These natural sweeteners work just as well in your coffee as in your family's favorite cookies or cakes, an important concern among my kids, whose sense of food—its color and taste—has been distorted by the artificial foods that are so heavily advertised.

You will be hard-pressed to find another book as complete as *The Green Kitchen Handbook*. It tells you not only how to stock your pantry so as to create ecologically friendly, healthier meals, but also how to compost without smells or mess, and how to make your own cheap, safe cleaning products that really work. It's the kitchen aid of all kitchen aids.

Bringing our lives into better balance with nature—reducing and reusing, eating organic, composting—depends on our making lots of little changes. What sounds so simple can oftentimes be quite difficult if you don't know where to start or lack the proper tools to introduce change. *The Green Kitchen Handbook* is that rare book filled with all the missing pieces, the essential details, and the once-inherited-but-nearly-forgotten know-how that will make those big life changes much easier and more fun to make.

My work takes me away from home a fair amount. This may be why it's so important to me that my home, especially my kitchen, reflect my values and help me live in a way that is ecologically responsible. My green kitchen serves both my family's needs and my own by providing all of us a place where we can replenish our energy and find repose. I am grateful to own a copy of *The Green Kitchen Handbook*; it is a clear guide to a safer, saner, simpler kitchen—the heart of the home.

Meryl Streep

Preface

It's a beautiful spring day. I've been out in the garden, where I proudly examined my new corn shoots and yanked last year's potatoes from the spinach bed and the cabbage patch they had invaded. Later, I'll return to pick some young lettuce leaves for dinner. I haven't been a gardener for long—just a few years really—but I'm hooked. It's changed what I eat, how I cook, and how I think about food.

No doubt I was ready to change, as many of us are. Beyond what people have learned about the importance of good health and fitness, we have become increasingly aware and concerned about the toll industrial food production has taken on the environment and our health. An educated consumer now must make food choices that not only enhance our health but also contribute to the protection of our natural resources. We want our food to be produced in ways that are "sustainable"—ways that reduce our dependence on costly inputs like pesticides and fuel, regenerate the growing environments for future generations, and respect and nourish those involved in its production.

With this in mind, Mothers & Others for a Livable Planet, the national nonprofit education organization working to promote responsible consumer choices that are safe and ecologically sustainable for this generation and the next, created *Eight Simple Steps to the New Green Diet,* a brief guide to help in planning our families' diets and making healthier, greener food choices. The steps were adapted from the research and writings of renowned nutritionists Joan Gussow, professor emeritus of nutrition and education at Teachers College, Columbia University (retired 1995), and Kate Clancy, professor of nutrition and food service management at Syracuse University. Both of them have dedicated their careers to advancing responsible eating and responsible food production.

The Green Kitchen Handbook is a simple extension of our eight steps. We want to help people integrate the New Green Diet and ecological principles into their daily lives—what they eat, how they shop, and how they manage their kitchens. We wrote *The Green Kitchen Handbook* to answer the many questions that arise— whether we live in a city, suburb, or country—when we make fundamental changes to what we eat. What are the components of a truly sustainable diet? Where are the best places to buy ecologically grown foods? Should I restock my pantry? With what? What about my freezer? Do I have to have a garden? How do I best deal with kitchen waste? What home-processing techniques might I try that will save me time and money?

In *The Green Kitchen Handbook,* we provide advice on all these matters and more, including seasonal menu planning, buying in bulk, shopping by mail order, packaging herb blends, cooking from scratch, composting, and eliminating packaging or trips to the store. *The Green Kitchen Handbook* also contains many surprises— including money- and time-budgeting ideas perfectly suited to a green lifestyle—that we came across in our research.

As the twentieth century comes to a close, the green diet is coming of age. The informed consumer is challenging the conventional wisdom, promoted by the multinational food companies, that food should be prepared without fuss, mess, or preparation time, and be quickly eaten. Consumers now recognize the trade-offs in health problems as well as damage to the environment. Responsible eating is important to good health. Fresh fruits and vegetables are widely available. And organic food, grown by certified farmers who employ ecological farming methods and only a limited set of synthetic pesticides, is now high on the grocery list.

People also are choosing to eat fewer and smaller portions of animal products, for health and environmental reasons. They are buying more local produce, shopping at farmers' markets, or joining a community-supported agriculture group (CSA). Keeping local farmers in the business of growing our food provides us all with many benefits in addition to providing fresher food. The most obvious is scenic countrysides. Other benefits include the maintenance of rural communities and lifestyles, and the use of less fuel and fewer postharvest pesticides for food transport and storage.

Great food from a green kitchen nourishes the soul as well as the body. Microwave dinners may be convenient, but they are not likely to replace the pleasing aromas and rich flavors of homemade meals made from locally grown sources. Nor can they serve to connect us to the earth, the seasons, the people who grow our food, and the places in which it grew. As our friend Alice Waters, chef and founder of Chez Panisse restaurant in California, has said, "Food can be transformative in everyone's life. . . . How you eat and how you choose your food is an act that combines the political—your place in the world of other people—with the most intensely personal—the way you use your mind and your senses, together for the gratification of your soul."

Let food transform your life, turn on your senses, and gratify your soul. May *The Green Kitchen Handbook* be your guide.

Wendy Gordon
Executive Director
Mothers & Others for a Livable Planet

Acknowledgments

I'd like to thank Mothers & Others for a Livable Planet for teaching me so much about sustainable agriculture. In particular I thank Wendy Gordon, Betsy Lydon, and Lisa Lefferts for reading the manuscript with care. And I will be forever indebted to Meryl Streep, cofounder of Mothers & Others, for writing such a lovely foreword.

A heartfelt thanks to all the friends and family who slogged through the early drafts and offered valuable insights: Daniel Berthold-Bond (my steadfastly supportive husband, who read every word of every draft), Nancy Prosser (my mother, who has taught so many to care about our natural world), Susan Harp, Fara Shaw Kelsey, Jenny Spenser, and Carl Frankel. Thanks, too, to Rachel Cavel for her help, Jenny Spenser for the research she did as a most generous and committed volunteer, Sandy and Dick Collins, and Erin Schulman. I am also indebted to Joan Gussow, Fred Kirschenmann, and Deborah Lee for generously offering their expertise; and Spectrum Naturals, a manufacturer of cooking and medicinal oils, which provided invaluable information on oils for chapter 4.

Last but not least I want to thank my agent, Lisa Ross, and my editor at HarperCollins, Jennifer Griffin. Their professional grace and Jennifer's deft editorial hand added a great deal to the pleasure of writing *The Green Kitchen Handbook*.

Introduction

Mi Taku Oyaku. (We are all interconnected.)

—Lakota Prayer

The kitchen is the center of our homes—like the center of a wheel, around which all revolves. From quiet family suppers to cooking for a party, activities in our kitchens are as multidimensional as those of us who inhabit them. The kitchen is also the center of a greater community, the hub from which many connections radiate to the world at large. Like the spokes of a wheel linking the center to the rim, the kitchen and community are interconnected in everyday life when we bring things in (such as groceries) and take things out (such as garbage).

The practical decisions we make regarding our kitchens may seem mundane at first glance—what kinds of food we buy and whom we buy them from—yet the impact of these choices affects our health and the health of our communities. In return, the practical decisions of the community affect the health of our families. If we buy food from an industrial farm that pollutes the water, that polluted water may enter our own kitchen, or that of a friend or family member many miles away. If a community allows the use of excessive packaging, then when that packaging becomes garbage it can contaminate our homes from incinerator ash and as leachate from landfills.

Making responsible choices for the kitchen according to their impact on the health of our friends and family, the health of the community, and ultimately the earth, is the process that leads to establishing a green kitchen. This book gives you the tools to make positive choices about the kinds of foods you choose to eat, how you prepare them, where you can find sustainable farms that grow and produce the food, and how you can set up and maintain an ecological kitchen. Achieving a green kitchen takes time; don't expect to make all the changes overnight. But once you start the process, you may find that the feeling of centering and interconnectedness it gives you urges you to continue.

BRINGING IT ALL BACK HOME

You may be wondering how it will be possible to incorporate such changes into your everyday life. Putting philosophical principles into practice is all well and good on paper, you might say, but you have hardly enough time to get dinner on the table, not to mention overhaul the kitchen. Let us assure you of one very important thing—a green kitchen can actually bring simplicity to your life.

Learning why and how to make the best "green" choices takes some time, but it becomes easier. Once you start putting the principles into practice, and have learned the tools and skills you need, a green kitchen takes no more time to maintain than any other kind of kitchen—and it may take less. A green kitchen can be a gourmet kitchen, a traditional American kitchen, any kind of kitchen, but one thing it does not need to be is complicated. In fact, as you will soon learn, if you have a well-stocked pantry, make a quick trip to the market once a week for fresh food, and reduce your garbage as much as possible, then you can conveniently maintain a green kitchen.

Your food choices may or may not change much, depending on how you eat now. The greenest kitchen is one stocked with real food—unprocessed and unrefined as much as possible, and freshly picked and locally produced when available. It features kitchen counters resplendent with such local fruit as strawberries, melons, and pears, and a refrigerator full of just-picked seasonal vegetables, like sugar snap peas, available from a community farm. The days when a meal of whole foods consisted of a bowl of grains that tasted like sawdust went out with the sixties. Whole food now means fresh and flavorful, tasting real, not of chemicals. A salad is a rich diversity of greens, dessert is an organic fruit sorbet with fruit juice used as a sweetener.

Quinoa and the rattlesnake bean are examples of some new foods you can explore here. (Actually, they are ancient, but new to most Americans.) Chapter 4, "The Green Pantry," gives you a tour of such delicious but lesser-known foods. There are also some less commonly used tools you will be introduced to in this book—appliances that are particularly helpful for processing whole grains and nuts. Chapter 6, "The Ecological Kitchen," provides details.

The Green Kitchen Handbook helps you avoid food that is overly packaged and processed. Prepackaged food is not the time-saving bargain it may appear. Take the simple example of oatmeal. Our choices are the one-minute prepackaged-by-serving type, or real oats, which may take five minutes to cook. In preparing breakfast, what difference does it make if the oats take five minutes rather than one to cook? If we choose the five-minute oatmeal, not only is the taste incomparably better, but there is also less packaging for the garbage . . . and it really doesn't take any more of *our* time.

This book is also designed to address some of the worries that nag us when we think about food. Should we worry about pesticides in our children's food? If so, is there an affordable way to replace conventional food with organic? What food additives should we avoid whenever possible? If we are concerned about cleaning our kitchens with toxic chemicals, what are we supposed to use instead?

This book will help put your good intentions into practice. It can help you take charge of your family's nutritional health. And in so doing, it will give you a feeling of peace and accomplishment.

FOOD CHOICES: THE NEW GREEN DIET

Periodically, the U.S. Department of Agriculture (USDA) and the U.S. Department of Health and Human Services (USDHHS) publish Dietary Guidelines for Americans. The guidelines are designed to offer expert nutritional advice to help answer consumers'

Dietary Guidelines for Americans

🌿 Eat a variety of foods.

🌿 Maintain healthy weight.

🌿 Choose a diet low in fat, saturated fat, and cholesterol.

🌿 Choose a diet with plenty of vegetables, fruits, and grain products.

🌿 Use sugars only in moderation.

🌿 Use salt and sodium only in moderation.

🌿 If you drink alcoholic beverages, do so in moderation.

(Source: U.S. Department of Agriculture and the U.S. Department of Health and Human Services; Third Edition, 1990.)

questions about what we should eat for a well-balanced diet. To aid in understanding the guidelines, the USDA compiled the Food Guide Pyramid as an outline for consumers to use for figuring out what to eat each day based on the Dietary Guidelines.

While the Dietary Guidelines give what most experts consider sound nutritional advice, the recommendations don't consider the impact the food choices have on the environment. They also don't

FOOD GUIDE PYRAMID
A Guide to Daily Food Choices

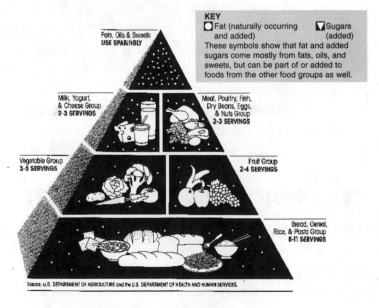

address issues of concern about artificial additives and pesticides, or food artificially manipulated by bioengineering, or irradiation. The New Green Diet is a set of guidelines developed by Mothers & Others for a Livable Planet that combines the Dietary Guidelines for Americans with advice that addresses environmental concerns.

The genesis for much of the New Green Diet is found in a 1986 article published in the *Journal of Nutrition Education* titled "Dietary Guidelines for Sustainability" by Joan Dye Gussow, professor emeritus of nutrition and education at Teachers College, Columbia University (retired 1995), and Kate Clancy, professor of nutrition and food service management at Syracuse University. Gussow and Clancy argued in the introduction that the environmental implications of our food choices need to be addressed. Farmers' dependency on cheap fossil fuels needs to be analyzed, and sustainable agriculture needs to be heralded because it is a system "that uses human and natural resources to produce food and fiber in a manner that is conservative, that is, in a manner that is not wasteful of such finite resources as top-soil, water, and fossil energy." Finally, food choices need to be judged on how much energy was required to produce them.

Drawing from "Dietary Guidelines for Sustainability," Wendy Gordon, Mothers & Others' executive director, and other staff elaborated on the guidelines, making them more specific in their support of sustainable agriculture and healthful food choices. Eight steps were defined to help put the New Green Diet into practice. Chapter 2 offers detailed information on why and how to follow these eight steps.

Eight Steps to the New Green Diet

1. Eat organic food.
2. Eat locally grown food.
3. Eat seasonal food.
4. Eat a variety of food.
5. Eat low on the food chain.
6. Eat whole foods with adequate fiber.
7. Avoid processed food.
8. Reduce packaging.

If we follow the recommendations shown in USDA's Food Guide Pyramid, say in eating two to four servings of fruit, and also choose the fruit according to the steps of the New Green Diet, we will choose fruit that has been grown on a sustainable farm, a farm that caretakes the earth. The fruit will have been grown locally, so that the least possible amount of energy is used to transport it to our tables. The fruit possibly may also be an unusual kind of fruit— an Arkane or Molly's Delicious apple, for example—grown from an heirloom seed to help protect biodiversity. It will not have been irradiated or bioengineered, and will be minimally packaged.

Following the New Green Diet is not complicated. Just-picked, juicy, ripe, local, organic food such as tomatoes or peaches that may be overflowing from bushel baskets at farm stands or farmers' markets are incomparably superior to the seasonless and flavorless fare of watery cucumbers, gas-ripened and colorless tomatoes, bland broccoli, and tasteless red peppers commonly available. And as anyone who has experienced the flavor and color of an egg laid that morning from a local neighbor's hen knows, factory eggs don't compare to those from small, local farms, nor does the flavor of meat full of antibiotics and hormones compare to that of organic meat.

FOOD SOURCES: SUSTAINABLE AGRICULTURE

How we eat determines to a considerable extent how the world is used.

—Wendell Berry, farmer and author

Making choices about where and how our food is grown and produced is one of the most important transitions in the process of achieving a green kitchen. There are many reasons for this. Sustainable farms nourish on a number of levels: they provide wholesome foods grown without synthetic chemicals in healthy soil, and the farms caretake the environment in our local communities and the larger community of which we are all a part.

Organic farmer Fred Kirschenmann is one of sustainable agriculture's most eloquent spokespeople. Kirschenmann received a Ph.D. in philosophy from the University of Chicago, but his devotion to sustainable farming practices compelled him to become a farmer full-time at the Kirschenmann Family Farm in Medina, North Dakota. He is the president of Farm Verified Organic and on the board of directors of Mothers & Others.

Above all, Kirschenmann believes supporting sustainable farms is of value for our communities. Observing that many view organic agriculture *only* as a safer food source, it is not given the importance it deserves. Organic farms should be recognized, Kirschenmann believes, for having a positive impact on the environment, soil quality, and the ecology of neighborhoods. "It is important to understand that what we are involved in here is a fundamentally different way of producing food, which has important social and political consequences for us all." Far more than just providing safe food, eating organic food supports a more ecologically sound way of eating.

In Kirschenmann's view, industrial farming upsets ecological balances and attempts to totally control nature. To accomplish this, industrial farms rely heavily on cheap, nonrenewable fossil fuel. Producing, transporting, processing, and marketing the food all depend heavily on it. In fact, without cheap fuel, industrial agriculture would be impossible because it would be too expensive. But Kirschenmann believes we will use up the earth's stores of oil sometime in the next century. What will happen to industrial agriculture then?

Organic farms use 70 percent less energy than conventional, industrial farming practices, according to a study at North Dakota State University. Recycling nutrients, careful ecological management, and using natural ecological balances to solve pest problems are the reasons for less energy use, Kirschenmann thinks. Being aware of the interactions among the soil fauna, wildlife, native plant species, and the climate help make an ecosystem work in a healthy way. Large routinized industrial farms, where one size fits all, can't function this way. In contrast to working for the health of the soil and wildlife, industrial farming actually contaminates groundwater and has resulted in the loss of over half of the nation's topsoil.

"What we haven't taken into account is the hidden costs of this food system. One of the costs is environmental . . . and it hasn't been accounted for and paid for." Kirschenmann laments the damage to the land, believing firmly that food can be produced without spoiling the environment and using up the earth's precious resources. "Organic agriculture emerged because a few farmers simply didn't go along with the attempt to industrialize agriculture. Instinctively they felt that an agriculture that sought to bind, gag, and blindfold nature and render her helpless, was the wrong path."

Choosing to buy food from sustainable farms supports a healthy ecological neighborhood. Farmer Laura Freeman, of Laura's Lean Beef, a sustainable farm in Lexington, Kentucky, observes,

The most important force in the sustainable agriculture movement is you: the person who shops for food. Farmers, after all, are in the food business. It is this link—between farmers and people who eat—that we are working so hard to repair. . . . You'd be surprised at how much influence you have.

As consumers we can help establish local outlets for sustainable farms. We can change the stores we shop at, and change the sorts of farms that supply them. The story of Bread Alone Bakery, in Woodstock, New York, provides an inspiring success story of how wholesome food can be brought into the mainstream. This bakery, located in the Catskill Mountains, makes organic, whole grain bread in wood-fired French ovens. The local community ate so much of this delicious bread so enthusiastically that the company has grown big enough to provide bread to all the local supermarkets. In this one small town people's support of a local baker was influential in having some of the food sold in local supermarkets replaced by a more sustainable kind. And by supporting the local baker, they were in turn able to support the organic farm that provided the grain. Change toward a more sustainably grown food supply is in our hands.

Woodstock is not alone. No matter where you live in the country, there are simple ways to find whole, organic food. Chapter 3 provides details about how to find fresh organic food at farmers' markets, community-supported agriculture, food co-ops, subscription farms, farm stands, green supermarkets, health food stores, and even traditional supermarkets.

Once you start eating locally grown organic produce, it is hard to give it up. If you don't already, you may be inspired to start "putting it by." Chapter 4, "The Green Pantry," provides information on how to preserve the foods of the harvest so you can enjoy them throughout the year. There are directions for how to freeze, can, dry, and even store in a cold cellar. In fact, you may get so inspired by the attributes of fresh produce that you may want to start growing your own.

PUTTING IT ALL TOGETHER: THE SECRETS OF SUCCESS

Once you have established sources of good, year-round, local organic food—one of the more difficult challenges for many of us, depending on where in the country we live—a green kitchen becomes a place of simplicity and convenience. If we allow seasonal, local food to determine our menus, half our work is done. No more trying to conjure something up out of the seasonless fare of produce we are all so tired of.

If we let the earth's current harvest be our guide, we hardly need to give a thought to menus. Just think of pies, for instance. If strawberries and rhubarb are showing up in local farms, it seems like time for a strawberry rhubarb pie. A few weeks later it may be blackberry and raspberry season, and then time for mountain blueberries. Before we have time to get bored with the berries we'll have moved on to peaches and pears and apples, then pumpkin and quince. By late winter, apple and pumpkin may be a bit commonplace, but just when we tire of them, up pop the strawberries and rhubarb again.

Main dishes may be a little bit more complex to conjure up from what is locally available, but not much. Cooking from scratch comes in very handy here. A few basic pasta dishes can carry us throughout the year in style: pasta and peas in the spring, pasta with fresh tomatoes and zucchini in the summer, pasta and sun-dried tomatoes in the winter: the combinations are endless. These menus also take very little time to prepare. If we draw a blank, however, we can always flip through the index of our favorite cookbooks for inspiration. From A for *asparagus,* to Y for *yams,* cookbooks are full of produce-specific ideas for menus.

If we allow our taste buds to savor the full flavor of freshly picked vegetables and fruit, we naturally begin to turn away from packaged and processed food by choice. Having a well-stocked pantry is the missing link to making a green kitchen convenient, and once you have one, you will always want one; it makes life so much calmer! No more rushed trips to the store because you are out of something. If you have grains, nuts and seeds, oils, spices, flours, herbs, and teas on hand, with the addition of a few fresh vegetables, you can easily put meals together on the spot. Little shopping, little fuss. As you get more proficient at cooking according to what's seasonally available, you can shop once a month for the pantry, and make one quick trip out each week for fresh food.

Maintaining the kitchen as a healthful and holistic place is another process that is addictive. Once you have successfully cleaned the oven without dizzying fumes, it is *very* hard to go back. Clean air and water are not difficult to ensure in a kitchen, but you need some skills and tools to do so. Cleaning and controlling pests without toxic synthetic chemicals is a very easy and positive way to make a difference in indoor air quality. Reducing garbage by composting and recycling is another satisfying task. Chapter 6, "The Ecological Kitchen," offers tips and advice for cleaning, pest control, and more.

Just as a sustainable farm nourishes on a number of levels, so too does a green kitchen. Conserving water, recycling, minimizing garbage, and making sustainable food choices—they all benefit our families as well as the community. Communities are made up of individuals. If enough of us establish green kitchens we will end up helping our communities progress toward a sustainable future, benefiting us all.

The New Green Diet

STEP 1: EATING ORGANICALLY PRODUCED FOOD

The term *organic* refers to how food has been grown and processed. Organic food is produced on farms that work to build an ecological partnership with nature. They replenish and maintain soil fertility, build a biologically diverse agriculture, and don't rely on the use of synthetic pesticides and fertilizers.

Organic agriculture strives toward being sustainable—*sustainable* meaning that which can be continued indefinitely, without depletion of resources beyond a rate such that they could be renewed. It is an approach to farming where all effort is made to maintain the farm ecosystem in a healthy balance. The ultimate goal of organic agriculture is to protect the health of the environment at large, including that of people, plants, and animals.

Almost everyone reports that organic food is dramatically more flavorful than food from industrialized farms. Well-balanced soil supports strong, healthy plants; it makes sense that such plants taste better. Organic food is usually minimally processed and contains no artificial ingredients.

THE MEANING OF CERTIFIED ORGANIC

The Organic Foods Production Act (OFPA) of 1990, to be implemented in 1997, is a law that requires the USDA to establish a national organic certification program to define *organic* and to regulate the organic foods production industry. Under the OFPA law, all organic certification agencies will be accredited by the USDA.

If a food is labeled "certified organic," under the new law you will be guaranteed that the product has been verified to have been grown and handled according to specific procedures and guidelines (highlighted below). Certified organic food also meets all federal, state, and local health requirements.

ORGANIC AGRICULTURE

Farming techniques used in organic agriculture are designed to work with the ecosystem of the farm as a whole. Organic farmer Fred Kirschenmann observes,

[Organic agriculture] seeks to cooperate with nature, rather than control nature. Productivity is achieved through nutrient recycling that attends to the health of the whole soil system, rather than spiking the soil with a few nutrients. It seeks to maintain and enhance the natural eco-logical balances of nature, rather than controlling a few species of pests. It seeks to align itself with the natural ecologies and evolutionary processes of the place in which the farm existed, rather than artificially dividing nature into camps of good species and bad species. As the word "organic" implies, it seeks to integrate the parts of the system into a healthy balanced whole.

Industrial farming is very energy-intensive. It has been docu-mented that organic farming, on the other hand, reduces energy use by 70 percent. "This energy conservation was achieved not by substituting natural inputs for synthetic ones, but by recycling nutrients to maintain fertility, and using natural ecological balances to solve pest problems." Kirschenmann believes that industrial farming is only possible because of cheap oil prices and huge gov-ernment subsidies.

The United States is facing the worst topsoil erosion in history due to its current agricultural practices of chemical-intensive, mono-crop farming. The U.S. Soil Conservation Service estimates over three billion tons of topsoil are eroded from U.S. croplands each year—twenty-five billion tons globally. "We've lost well over one half of our topsoil, and most of that has been just in the last seventeen years," laments Kirschenmann.

However, he observes that "the damage to farmland from conventional farming is reversible by implementing sustainable farming practices." For more on the differences between industrial agriculture and organic agriculture, see chapter 1.

Farms that sell certified organic food are inspected annually and need to provide certifiers with a written plan of their organic management techniques. Farmers must provide detailed records of diversity on their farms, fertility practices for the replenishing of soil, recycling of materials and resources from within the farm, and the humane treatment of their farm animals. In order to be certified, agricultural products must have been grown on land that has gone through a three-year transition period when no substances prohibited for organic certification have been used.

Pesticides and Other Chemicals

Most of the synthetic chemicals used on industrial farms are prohibited from use on food that is to be certified as organic. Deciding which chemicals will be allowed for use on organic products is a hotly debated issue on the agenda of the National Organic Standards Board (NOSB), the group of national experts writing the law. Overall, however, the use of most synthetic chemicals is prohibited in the growing, processing, and handling of organic foods. This includes the majority of agricultural pesticides, herbicides, fungicides, and fertilizers. The chemicals that are allowed are those that have been deemed to be not harmful to health or the environment by the NOSB and are detailed on the National List of Permitted Synthetic Substances.

The reduction in the amount of chemicals used to produce certified organic food compared to conventional is profound. Prohibited chemicals are banned not only from crops but also from areas where the food is stored and even from the cleaning products used in the vicinity of the food. The barns that house livestock cannot be treated with prohibited pesticides.

Certified organic food cannot be called pesticide-free.

Pesticides have been found in isolated areas of the globe where no pesticides are used, drifting there from thousands of miles away. Organic certification does not mean these residues do not exist.

One of the most significant reasons to eat organic food, besides supporting organic agriculture, is to reduce the amount of agricultural pesticides used. The reasons for this are to protect human health, not the least of which is that of farmworkers, and to protect the environment.

PESTICIDES

The United States uses more agricultural pesticides than any other country in the world. According to the U.S. Environmental Protection Agency (EPA), 1.2 billion pounds of pesticides were used in the United States in 1995. The EPA figures only include active ingredients, not the "inert" chemicals that can comprise more than 50 percent of formulated pesticides, and wood preservatives and disinfectants. Where there is pesticide spray, there is also pesticide drift. Less than 0.1 percent of pesticides applied to crops reach the pest targeted, Cornell University scientist David Pimental reports. The rest goes into the air, into our streams and rivers, onto living organisms, or elsewhere on the earth. When the amount is in the billions of pounds there are serious consequences.

As told in *Our Stolen Future,* wildlife around the world are experiencing disruption of their normal hormonal patterns and immune systems, and pesticides are high on the list of chemicals thought to be responsible. Fish, frogs, and other aquatic animals eat or absorb persistent pesticides in waterways, which can affect them and other organisms that feed on them. Some pesticides concentrate in the tissues of organisms, causing the biggest problems in animals at the top of the food chain, such as birds, fish, and even people.

PESTICIDES AND HEALTH

The EPA has regulated pesticides according to whether they are cancer-causing substances or not. Despite some regulations, the list of pesticides that are possible or probable carcinogens is extensive.

Of the pesticides legally allowed to be used on food crops, the EPA considers 60 percent of the registered herbicides, 90 percent of the fungicides, and 30 percent of the insecticides to be potentially carcinogenic. Thirty-six pesticides that are known to cause cancer are now being phased out of use, and forty-nine more are being considered for removal. U.S. Food and Drug Administration (FDA) studies show that many pesticide violations (a violation results when higher residues are found on the produce than are legally allowed) are from pesticides and herbicides that are used illegally. But risk of cancer, while bad enough, is not the whole story.

A growing array of mysterious ailments reported by Gulf War veterans has been linked to the synergistic effect of small doses of different pesticides. Researchers at the University of Texas and Duke University found that when small amounts of organophosphate pesticides (amounts considered harmless) were used in combination in studies on chickens, they caused serious nerve damage. When two or more organophosphate pesticides were given to chickens, they caused brain and nerve damage. When three kinds of pesticides were given to chickens, many died. When one single pesticide was tested, there were no symptoms. The Gulf War veterans were exposed to small amounts of a number of different organophosphate pesticides—also called cholinesterase inhibitors—during the war. Many similar organophosphate pesticides are used in agriculture.

The immune system may also be at risk from pesticide exposure, according to research on pesticide use in developing countries by the World Resources Institute. The organization claims that there is a "large body" of evidence suggesting that pesticides can alter the immune system's normal structure, disregulate and disturb immune responses, and reduce immune resistance. One of the researchers, Dr. Robert Repetto, says that this weakening of the immune system may be "the most widespread public health threat from pesticides."

Some pesticides also can disrupt hormones and either mimic or block the action of naturally occurring hormones at various receptor sites throughout the body. When two or more hormone-disrupting pesticides are combined, their potency may jump a thousandfold, according to new studies. Pesticide residues are found in fruits, vegetables, fish, meats, and dairy products, as are other endocrine-disrupting chemicals such as PCBs and dioxins. Interestingly, a letter in the prestigious medical journal the *Lancet,* noted that members of the Danish Organic Farmers' Association had a "significantly higher" sperm density when compared with three groups of blue-collar workers. The organic farmers, when asked about their consumption of dairy products, reported that over half of their consumption was from organic sources.

The EPA has found 132 different pesticides in the groundwater of forty-five states, finding agriculture the largest cause. A recent study by the Environmental Working Group and Physicians for Social Responsibility noted that drinking water is commonly contaminated with two or more of the five major agricultural herbicides (atrazine, cyanazine, simazine, alachlor, and metolachlor). People living in small rural communities receive the greatest exposures because of runoff of pesticides from farmland into the water supply. Fish living in the contaminated lakes and streams will store some herbicides in their fat, bringing herbicides onto the dinner table.

Children are particularly vulnerable to possible harm from pesticides. A distinguished National Academy of Science study, *Pesticides in the Diets of Infants and Children* (June 1993), reported that the federal government takes a one-size-fits-all approach to the regulation of pesticides, even though infants and children have different growth rates and diets than do adults. Today's regulatory system does not consider that children's bodies may react differently to foreign substances. As a result, some children may be ingesting unsafe amounts of pesticides.

In addition to several case reports of childhood cancers following the use of pesticides in the home and yard, five separate studies have found a link between childhood exposure to pesticides and cancer, including leukemia and brain cancers. One study published in the *Journal of the National Cancer Institute* found that children whose parents used pesticides in the garden were six times as likely to develop leukemia as controls. While the exposures from food are much less intense than those received by directly applying pesticides, these studies taken collectively raise a red flag about pesticides and their role in some childhood cancers.

THE COST OF CERTIFIED ORGANIC FOOD

There is no way around it, certified organic produce and animal products cost more than nonorganic. There is one big exception to this rule, however, and that is certified organic packaged food. The prevailing opinion, that organic packaged food is more expensive than conventional, name brand food, is a misconception. In fact, Mothers & Others has found that organic meals, not including fresh produce, are actually comparably priced to meals prepared with conventional products. Some organic food—cheese, for example—does indeed cost a bit more than its conventional counterpart, but the organic crackers you might put the cheese on are significantly cheaper than conventional crackers. The prices average out over a day's worth of meals.

Although it costs a bit more to buy most certified organic produce and meat, when you buy organic food you are not passing any of the cost along to future generations, as happens when you buy food from many other farms. You could say that when you pay more for organic food, you are buying futures in the environment. There are many hidden environmental costs of industrialized farming that we pay for years after we leave the checkout counter. "Sustainable farms pay the full cost in this generation now, whereas factory farms charge some of their expense to the next generation," declares David Podoll, an organic turkey farmer from Prairie Road Organic Farm in North Dakota.

CERTIFIED ORGANIC PRODUCE

There can be a difference in appearance between organic and conventional produce. Organic produce may vary in size, be less uniform in shape or coloring, or may be mottled or blemished. Chemicals in conventional agriculture can be used for cosmetic purposes—to enhance coloring, firmness, roundness, and thickness of skin—and not just to fight bugs or fungus. A Cornell researcher estimates that from 10 to 20 percent of insecticides and fungicides are applied simply to comply with strict cosmetic standards. Organic produce is more perishable than conventional. It's also generally picked closer to ripeness, therefore apparently reducing its shelf life. For example, lettuce, tomatoes, and beans should be eaten within a few days of purchase. Slightly wilted produce, however, can be perked up by soaking it in cold water. One should be able to keep storable foods—potatoes, apples, beets, oranges, grapefruits, sweet potatoes—for a month or more in the refrigerator without any problem, whether these foods are organic or conventional. But be careful to check for molds; they can form on fruits during long-term storage. The skin of an organic orange may dry out more quickly than a conventional orange peel. It may not look as good as a result. But cut into it—even if it's been in your refrigerator for a while, it may still be incredibly juicy and tasty.

ORGANIC MEAT, DAIRY PRODUCTS, AND EGGS

At the time this book is being written, meat and poultry are by law not labeled as organically produced. Some states have organic livestock standards, however, and you can find out if the farm producing the meat adheres to them. Look for certified organic meat once the National Organic Standards take effect. But buying certified organic meat and dairy products grown in the United States will not protect you from contaminants in our land and water such as dioxin and PCBs that are eaten by livestock and stored in their fat. Buying certified organic meat, dairy products, and eggs, however, protects you from a host of other contaminants.

ORGANIC MEAT AND DAIRY PRODUCTS

Animal Is Fed Organic Feed and Allowed to Free-Range
Numerous reports indicate that animals raised on organic feed are significantly more healthy, and in fact using organic feed may be the first step a farmer can take to avoid having the healthy growth of his farm animals and produce depend on chemicals. In order to be considered organic by a certifying organization, the animals must be fed 100 percent certified organic feed, forage, and hay. Organic

feed is of benefit to you too because it does not contain pesticide residue, which you would be exposed to when you ate the animal or drank its milk. Poultry is allowed to free-range, allowing the birds to find food from a number of sources, providing a more well-rounded diet. Cows' pastures are rotated frequently, fertilizing the land as the cattle grazes and providing the cows with good, healthful grass to eat. The grazing area is never sprayed. Most animals that have been allowed to free-range are much more muscular than those that are confined, resulting in lower-fat meat. Last but not least, buying certified organic animal products helps ensure that the animals were raised humanely.

Animal Has Not Been Given Any Growth Stimulants or Antibiotics

Antibiotic residues can end up in meat. Animals raised on industrial farms receive on average up to thirty times more antibiotics than people do. The drugs are used not only to treat or prevent infections but also to make animals grow faster. Some antibiotics are becoming ineffective because of overuse. Much more virulent strains of bacteria, such as *E. coli* 0157:H7, have developed resistance to antibiotics. Animals that are sold as organic have never been treated with drugs.

ORGANIC EGGS

Organic eggs are from hens that have been raised on organic feed and have not been given antibiotics. Organic eggs are not necessarily fertile eggs—hens will lay eggs without ever even seeing a rooster. The word *free-range* is the best clue you have that the hens were raised in a more humane way. Large industrial laying hens are not allowed to free-range. Instead, they live indoors without exercise under twenty-four-hour lighting to confuse them into producing more eggs than is normal. Free-range hens are allowed outdoors, on the other hand, and have access to grubs and bugs, which help round out their diet. Some are allowed to live and mate with roosters according to their natural cycles.

ORGANIC STANDARDS AND YOUR OWN STANDARDS

There are a number of controversies that have developed around the details of particular organic standards. Can honey be considered organic even though it is impossible to control where bees collect pollen? How much organic food content must a processed product have in order to be labeled "organic" on the principal display panel? What chemicals are acceptable to use when the farmer is faced with a serious pest infestation? To ensure that certified organic food meets *your* standards, whatever the outcome of these controversies, contact the farm you buy your food from, or the farm's certifying agency. Doing this is easy with animal products such as meat and milk, as the packages are clearly labeled. It is less easy to identify the source of produce, but we recommend speaking with produce managers and asking them to supply you with information about the producers or certifying agencies.

STEPS 2 AND 3: EATING LOCAL, SEASONAL FOOD

We should be producing the fullest variety of foods to be consumed locally, in the countryside itself and in nearby towns and cities: meats, grains, table vegetables, fruits and nuts, dairy products, poultry and eggs. . . . We need . . . a system of decentralized, small-scale industries to transform the products of our fields and woodlands and streams: small creameries, cheese factories, canneries, grain mills, saw mills, furniture factories, and the like.

—Wendell Berry, farmer and author

Joan Gussow is among the first people who advocated eating locally and seasonally for environmental reasons. Now professor emeritus, in the 1980s she chaired the department of nutrition education at

Teachers College in New York City, and has written several books including *The Feeding Web* and *Chicken Little, Tomato Sauce and Agriculture*. She served as president of the Society for Nutritional Education, was a Chancellor's distinguished lecturer at the University of California, Berkeley, and was a member of the National Academy of Sciences committee linking diet and cancer.

Like most visionaries, Joan was viewed as highly unconventional when she first started talking about her ideas in the 1970s. They flew in the face of all the tenets of modern industrial agriculture. But Joan's views are ultimately based on enormous amounts of common sense. They have since been enthusiastically supported by the sustainable farming community.

Gussow first advocated eating locally in the late 1970s as a means of energy conservation. She observed that it takes a lot of gas and oil to transport food for thousands of miles, and it takes a lot more to keep it cold for all that distance. Locally produced food would not need to be refrigerated for such long periods of time nor would it need to be shipped. "I came to the conclusion that the only ecologically sound diet would be from foods available nearby, simply because of the transportation costs."

She believes there are other consequences of transporting food from many miles away, especially importing it from Third World countries. The reason it makes economic sense to ship the food is that the food is cheap (low labor costs) and transportation is cheap (low energy costs). But food is inexpensive from such countries because those who grow it are so poorly paid that they often can't afford to buy enough to eat for themselves. Energy costs are low, but the energy used is nonrenewable.

One big benefit of eating locally, Gussow believes, is that we see for ourselves how the land and water are treated by the farmers. The hidden costs of industrial agriculture, which the consumer usually doesn't see—overuse of water, chemicals, and loss of cropland, which ultimately threatens the food supply—would be right under our noses. The out-of-sight, out-of-mind mentality would necessarily change. Eating locally also will support local farmers and keep them skilled. Gussow believes that the underlying point is that "in the course of getting food for ourselves we must try to stop letting so many evils be done in our name in places we know nothing about."

Gussow eats a diet of local and seasonal produce herself, and has found this to be relatively easy. "We discovered to our great delight that not only could we feed ourselves almost exclusively from our garden, but in a quite surprising way eating local food in season actually grew on us." She and her husband work hard to preserve food, with a freezer and root cellar, and try to extend the seasons. The most difficult time, they find, is early April. Potatoes in the root cellar start getting soft and sprout, and the lettuce isn't up yet. Their diet follows what is available from their garden. They eat peas nonstop for six weeks or so, and then they don't eat them again until the same time the following year. They eat a lot of potatoes, onions, and garlic in the winter. They feel far from deprived: "Limits are a tonic to the human spirit. Look at the restrictions of haiku poetry, for example. Working within limits pushes your creativity," Gussow observes. In fact, Gussow believes deprivation is found instead in the same seasonless, regionless diet day after day that is produced by the industrial global supermarket.

Gussow asks people to make a list of things they really don't want to give up and that can't be produced locally. She says that it is surprising how small a list it is. Coffee is always on the list. (She tells them that coffee is okay for people to import as long as it is produced sustainably. Coffee does not weigh a lot and therefore costs less energy to transport, and it doesn't need to be refrigerated en route.) One person at a conference she attended added artichokes to the list, and a farmer announced that he was growing artichokes at his farm in Vermont!

Gussow urges growers to be inventive by extending the seasons and pushing the limits of what they can grow. She herself grows some citrus in her home north of New York City. She has lime and lemon trees, and even a grapefruit and an orange tree. Papaws— which are supposed to taste like bananas—can live in the north, and she is trying to grow them. She welcomes investigations to determine if local greenhouses use less energy than importing food from elsewhere, or if solar greenhouses can become a realistic way to grow large amounts of food. "Local freezing and food processing are what we really need. We could create a market for frozen local organic food."

A local, seasonal diet doesn't mean one can't maintain an ethnic diet that has been grown locally, Gussow says. Chinese who live in New York City have New Jersey farmers who grow their vegetables. People who move north from the tropics, for example, can easily grow or buy locally grown hot peppers. And culturally appropriate seasonings help a lot to make food taste more familiar.

EATING LOCALLY

How should we define *local*? According to Joan Gussow, this is almost impossible to answer, but the most commonsense principle to follow is that the fewer miles the food travels from the farm to your table, the better. (The average mouthful of food travels 1,200 miles from farm to factory to warehouse to supermarket to our plates. Much of it comes from countries many more thousands of miles away. The United States is the largest food importer in the world.)

Calculate the distance it takes to get the food to you, and choose the closest producers. Your town is closer than the far reaches of your state, for example; your state is closer than a farm two states over; if you live in the East, Florida is closer than California; if you live in the state of Washington, Florida is closer than Brazil, and so forth. No matter where you live, search out local farmers' markets whenever possible. Best of all, try starting a garden.

Some people are starting a "foodshed" movement, recommending that people buy all their food from sources within the area of one's community, defined much like a watershed. The foodshed would provide all the food in the region, exporting any surplus and importing a few exotics many can't do without, such as coffee. The foodshed movement certainly makes a lot of sense, and organic farmers would benefit because they would have to provide a wide diversity of crops to meet all the nutritional needs of their community. All farmers would benefit, as would the community, if the farmers tried to reduce pesticide use to protect the quality of local water.

Other organizations consider *local* to mean statewide. This approach works within the existing system; each state has a

Department of Agriculture, and these departments can become instrumental in working with farms, supermarkets, and consumers in their states, helping to interconnect them.

GETTING CHILDREN TO GO ALONG WITH IT

Do you live in northern Maine and have a child who loves pineapple, a fruit that grows in a tropical climate? What should you do about *that*? Martin Teitel provides wonderful advice through an analogy in *Rain Forest in Your Kitchen*.

For most people, regardless of religious belief, the end of December is a special time: decorations adorn stores, streets, and houses; aromas of fir trees, wood fires, and spiced cider waft through the air; special music, books, and clothes are brought out of closets. Would the holiday be as wonderful if we kept the Christmas tree up all year, opened presents every morning, or had turkey and stuffing for dinner each night? Hardly. Anticipation and memories are part of the magic of this time of year.

Boring old broccoli eaten night after night can be replaced instead with a gourmet menu changing from week to week according to what is being harvested. Sugar snap peas can be eaten in the spring, scallions in early summer, zucchini squash in August, sun-dried tomatoes in the fall. And, yes, pineapple as a treat for birthdays and special occasions, especially in the fall.

GETTING TO KNOW YOUR FARMER'S SEASON

Following a diet of the seasonal harvest is a joy. In the East, spring begins with sweet strawberries and tart rhubarb, a perfect combination; berries and melons in the summer; apples, pears, even peaches in the fall and winter. Apples can be placed in cold storage, still crisp, to carry one to early spring, when the strawberries come in. Vegetables follow a different pattern, starting with peas and spinach, and moving to parsnips and sweet potatoes for winter stews.

California and New York's harvests are quite different.

California's climate makes for a long growing season, and there is much that can be eaten during the winter months, compared to New York. However, New York has its treasures too, and those of us who live in the East love the changes of the seasons, as they bring a change of diet too. Following are seasonal harvest charts of California and New York. If you live somewhere in between the two states, follow the harvest calendar most closely resembling the food grown in your climate.

Seasonal Harvest Calendar for California

FRUIT

Spring
Avocados, bananas, cherries, grapefruit, lemons, mangoes, navel oranges, papaya, pineapple, plums, rhubarb, strawberries

Summer
Apricots, blueberries, boysenberries, cantaloupe, grapefruit, grapes, honeydew melons, lemons, nectarines, peaches, Persian melons, strawberries, Valencia oranges, watermelons

Fall
Apples, cantaloupe, cranberries, dates, grapefruit, grapes, honeydew melons, lemons, kiwi, papayas, pears, Persian melons, persimmons

Winter
Grapefruit, lemons, kiwi, navel oranges, persimmons, tangelos, tangerines

VEGETABLES

Spring
Artichokes, asparagus, broccoli, cabbage, cauliflower, celery, cucumbers, garlic, leeks, lettuce, mushrooms, onions, peas, potatoes, rhubarb, snap beans, spinach, squash, watercress

Summer
Artichokes, cabbage, carrots, cauliflower, celery, corn, cucumbers, eggplant, garlic, green peppers, kohlrabi, lettuce, mushrooms, okra, onions, potatoes, spinach, squash, tomatoes, watercress

VEGETABLES

Fall
Artichokes, broccoli, cabbage, carrots, cauliflower, celery, chili peppers, corn, cucumbers, dry beans, endive, escarole, green peppers, leeks, lettuce, onions, parsnips, peas, potatoes, squash, rutabaga, spinach, sweet potatoes, turnips

Winter
Artichokes, broccoli, brussels sprouts, carrots, cauliflower, celery, lettuce, mushrooms, potatoes, rutabaga, spinach, squash, tomatoes, turnips

HOW TO BUY LOCAL IN WINTER

Out-of-season produce is an extravagance because it is so energy-intensive to transport to your kitchen. In the winter we should all try to eat frozen, dried, and canned food, and that which comes out of local root cellars.

Eating frozen fruits and vegetables, especially from local producers, and that which comes out of local root cellars is your very best option during the winter months. Frozen foods retain much of their nutritional content, in addition to cutting energy costs in transportation. Dried and canned foods are also nutritious options.

The key to eating food that has been preserved in some way for the winter months is to buy it from local processors. Most frozen or canned packaged food will state who the processor and distributor are on the package. Let that address be your guide to help you determine if it is "local" or not. Most food is frozen on the West Coast because of the longer growing season. Food is frozen immediately in local processing plants after being picked, to retain the most nutritive qualities. However, East Coast processors do exist, and once you identify a brand, look for it whenever you shop. For more information on food-processing locations, contact the American Frozen Food Institute (1764 Old Meadow Lane, Suite 350, McLean, VA 22102) or the Canned Food Information Council

Seasonal Harvest Calendar for New York State

FRUIT

Late Spring

Rhubarb, strawberries

Summer

Blackberries, blueberries, boysenberries, cherries, currants, red raspberries, strawberries

Fall

Apples, cantaloupe, grapes, honeydew melons, peaches, pears, plums, quince, watermelons

Winter

Cold storage fruit: Apples, pears

VEGETABLES

Late Spring

Asparagus, mushrooms (cultivated), peas, spinach

Summer

Beans (snap), celery, corn, cucumbers, eggplant, endive, escarole, fennel, kale, kohlrabi, lettuce, mushrooms, onions, peppers, radishes, summer squash, tomatoes, watercress

Fall

Acorn squash, beans (dried), beets, broccoli, brussels sprouts, cabbage, carrots, cauliflower, celeriac, celery, corn, eggplant, garlic, jerusalem artichokes, kale, leeks, onions, parsnips, potatoes, pumpkin, rabe, rutabaga, winter squash

Winter

Vegetables from root cellars and cold storage, such as beets, cabbage, carrots, leeks, onions, parsnips, potatoes, pumpkins, sweet potatoes, turnips, winter squash

(500 North Michigan Avenue, Suite 200, Chicago, IL 60611).

For more on how to find local farms, see chapter 3, "The New Foragers: New Ways to Shop and Acquire Food."

STEP 4: EATING A VARIETY OF FOODS

We all need a broad range of nutrients for optimum health, and when we eat a wide *variety* of foods, this requirement is likely to be met. The wider the variety, the greater the chance of getting the nutrients we need, reports the FDA.

The USDA's Food Guide Pyramid is a good place to learn about food groups—grains, fruits, vegetables, protein, dairy products, and fats—and the recommended number of servings for each group. The USDA recommends eating four to six servings of grain dishes, two to four servings of fruit, three to five servings of vegetables, two to three servings of dairy products, two to three servings of protein, and no more than a small amount of fats, oils, and sweets each day. Within each food group there is a world of variety. By choosing variety within food groups and eating from each of the food groups every day, you obtain a wider range of nutritional variety and also support the growing of a wide genetic diversity of foods.

Oats, rye, barley, brown rice, buckwheat, quinoa, and spelt are just a few grains besides wheat that offer variety in the grain food category. Fruit can include apples, pears, plums, oranges, grapefruit, melons, and strawberries, as well as dried fruit such as apple rings. As you will see below, within a food type there can be many varieties. There are dozens of varieties of apples, for example. The world of vegetables offers everything from spring spinach to cucumbers to hearty fall pumpkins and squashes. Protein can be derived from beans such as black beans, pinto and navy beans, and nuts, not just from animal products. Dairy products, while not necessary if you are a vegan (see step 5), can include low-fat cottage cheese, Quark (a European spreadable cheese similar to cream cheese but without much fat), and milk.

Food companies in the United States offered 15,006 *new* food products in 1994, and this number increases each year. These new food products do not represent variety! Just a few species of plants— primarily corn, wheat, rice, and potatoes—provide 90 percent of our food. The hundreds of food products available in supermarkets are not made up of hundreds of kinds of plants, but just these few, rearranged in myriad different boxes and recipes.

While traditional agriculture depended on eighty thousand species of plants, industrial agriculture now provides most of the food on our planet from just fifteen to thirty species of cultivated plants. The National Academy of Sciences (NAS) has found that "nearly all plant-breeding programs in the U.S. emphasize yield, uniformity, market acceptability and pest resistance, but not nutritional quality." Indeed, breeding plants for the characteristics desirable for industrial production and marketing often lowers the plants' nutritional values.

VARIETY AND SUSTAINABLE FARMS

To keep an organic farm in a thriving natural balance, it is essential for the farmer to grow a wide variety and diversity of plants to keep the soil healthy. Because of the wide range of crops grown, however, the farm also has a wider range of types of food to sell. If the public will only eat a few commodities over and over again, there is no market for the organic farm's wider selection of produce. The farmer's industrial counterpart, on the other hand, will be monocropping—growing nothing but a few commodities—and while the market supports growing these few products, industrial farms can only grow them with the help of synthetic pesticides and fertilizers.

Buying a variety of local, seasonal food from organic farms helps support the farmer who plants a diversity of crop. Making the choice to support this variety grown on local, sustainable farms has far-reaching implications. Great damage is done to the planet's genetic resources when we rely so heavily on so few plant varieties. Martin Teitel points out in *Rain Forest in Your Kitchen* that farms in Chile, for example, have displaced their own native and traditional fruits and vegetables in favor of the same fifteen to thirty species of crops grown around the world. This threatens native crops with extinction.

WHAT'S AT STAKE: THE SEEDS OF LIFE

"The loss of genetic diversity—silent, rapid, inexorable—is leading us to a rendezvous with extinction, to the doorstep of hunger on a scale we refuse to imagine," writes Kenny Ausubel in *Seeds of Change: The Living Treasure*. Farmers and gardeners need not only to grow a wide variety of crops but also to choose the seeds they use with care. Choosing to use open pollinated and heirloom seeds that have been passed down through the millennia, instead of the commercially available F1 hybrids, is critical to avoiding conditions that can cause famine, according to Ausubel. He and other experts around the world contend that far from being a nostalgic movement, choosing a widely biodiverse variety of foods is critical to our future survival.

To understand this crisis—one in proportion to global warming and the ozone hole, according to many—we need to understand seeds, two kinds to be specific. One kind is called first-generation hybrids (F1 hybrids), which are hand pollinated, patented, often sterile, and genetically identical within food types and are sold from multinational seed companies. They have broad commercial appeal because they are absolutely uniform. The other kind of seeds is called heirloom or open-pollinated and have been passed on from generation to generation. With heirloom seeds there are ten thousand varieties of apples, compared to the very few F1 hybrid apple types. To illustrate the differences between these seed types, and the consequences of using each, let's follow two tomatoes—one from an F1 hybrid seed, and the other from an heirloom, open-pollinated seed—back from our dinner tables to the origin of the seed.

F1 HYBRID TOMATO

When you sit down to eat a salad with a tomato that you bought at a supermarket, chances are that the tomato was grown from an F1 hybrid seed. Though it is unlikely that when you were in the produce section you thought about the seed that grew your tomato, you may be very surprised to know that your F1 hybrid tomato came from a seed that is not found in nature.

Breeders make F1 hybrids by "selfing" plants—making them reproduce by using the plant's own pollen. The resulting seeds are genetically identical, a trait desirable for industrial farms, which grow thousands of acres of one kind of food. The seeds are bred for large-scale food production, prizing yield per acre, uniformity of color and consistency, and pest resistance.

There are a number of important problems hidden in the story of F1 hybrids. One is that F1 hybrid seeds have "hybrid vigor"— unusual productivity for the first-generation plant—after which their seeds tend to be sterile, or the plants are weak. Farmers have to buy new seeds every year, posing a serious problem for poor countries. Second, because the tomato you bought is most likely genetically identical to the tomato you will buy the next day and for the rest of the winter, you will not be getting a variety of nutritional benefits, as you would if you were eating different tomato types. Third, if all industrial farms around the country are growing F1 tomato plants, they are forcing out of the market the thousands of diverse tomato varieties that have, over the course of centuries, adapted to withstand drought, freezing, and blight.

OPEN-POLLINATED, HEIRLOOM TOMATOES

To find a tomato that is genetically unique you most likely would have to go to a farmers' market or grow your own. Food grown from heirloom and open-pollinated seeds has now become that obscure. But the seed that grew the tomato you went out of your way to buy or grow came from a seed passed down through countless generations. And at a farmers' market, you may be able to buy four or five tomatoes from different gene pools, giving you nutritional variety and a variety of tastes and flavors as well.

Open-pollinated seeds are constantly being modified in nature because the plants cross-pollinate with others in the locale, passing genes back and forth. The genes have been fine-tuned over centuries to a variety of climate and soil conditions, as well as adapting to blights and pests, making the plants uniquely capable of staving off a variety of threats. Seeds survived in this way for millennia before chemical sprays and fertilizers existed. Modern farmers who caretake heirloom seeds almost always grow them organically. Whereas often an heirloom seed will be native to a region, heirlooms do not necessarily imply native species—immigrants have brought their seeds to the United States for years, and the seeds have been domesticated.

When you add an heirloom tomato to your salad you will find it more flavorful than the uniform kind available at the supermarket. It may not look perfect, and may not even look like another tomato plucked from the same plant. Because of this, industrial farmers do not want to grow them, because they don't provide the uniformity or yield of F1 tomatoes. All the more reason to save this esoteric tomato's seeds, pass them on, and by doing so you may have saved a type of tomato from extinction. "As we collect seeds . . . we become aware of the part that the ancestors play in getting them to us. Then we have to be aware that we are the ancestors of the next stage," observes Kathleen Harrison, an associate of Seeds of Change, a company that sells heirloom seeds.

VULNERABILITY OF OUR FOOD SUPPLY

Unless we preserve diversity, our food supply is vulnerable. The Irish potato famine, which killed thousands of people and caused millions to emigrate in the 1840s, was caused by reliance on one kind of potato that turned out to be vulnerable to a fungus that grew in a damp spell. The fungus killed all of Ireland's potatoes. Because a biodiverse potato gene pool hadn't been saved, the main food source was wiped out for years until a blight-resistant potato was found in Peru many years later. A modern F1 hybrid potato seed would not have solved the problem in Ireland unless the particular seed had the gene against the blight, which is highly unlikely.

According to *Seeds of Change,* we now lose to oblivion three plant species an hour. Today, a blight-resistant alternative food source may no longer exist. Ausubel observes, "Of the cornucopia of reliable cultivated food plants available to our grandparents in 1900, today 97 percent are gone. Since the arrival of Columbus, 75 percent of native food plants have disappeared in the Americas." In modern times, when difficult blights and fungi attack their F1 hybrid plants, industrial farms use huge amounts of pesticides. Yet pesticide- and fungicide-resistant strains of plant diseases are developing all the time. The Irish famine could be a grim harbinger of things to come.

Two-thirds of the nearly five thousand nonhybrid vegetable varieties listed in the first *Garden Seed Inventory*, compiled by the Seed Savers Exchange in Iowa in 1985, were no longer available by 1994, according to the *New York Times*. Even more frightening is that of the thirteen to fourteen million species on earth, only about 13 percent have been identified, the *1995 Global Biodiversity Assessment* (Cambridge University Press), reports.

To do our part to protect biodiversity, we need to request local farmers and gardeners who sell at farmers' markets to offer us diverse foods. If they know there is a market, they may be more inclined to experiment with new species. Or, if you grow your own vegetables, choose open-pollinated and heirloom seeds, save the seeds yourselves, and pass them on to others.

The Mayan word *gene* means "spiral of life." The genes in the heirloom seeds give life to our future. Unless the 100 million backyard gardeners and organic farmers keep these seeds alive, they will disappear altogether. This is truly an instance where one person—a lone gardener in a backyard vegetable garden—can potentially make all the difference in the world.

Choosing a Variety of Diverse Foods to Protect Biodiversity

To give you some examples of genetically diverse foods, we have excerpted some plant descriptions from the *Bountiful Gardens Seed Catalog*. Published by Ecology Action and adapted/reprinted with kind permission of manager Bill Bruneau, the *Bountiful Gardens Seed Catalog* offers a number of open-pollinated and heirloom seeds. Ecology Action is a nonprofit organization committed to biointensive gardening methods. You can obtain a copy of the catalog by writing to Ecology Action, 5798 Ridgewood Road, Willits, CA 95490, or call 707-459-6410.

GREENS

Bronze Arrow Lettuce: A rare, long-standing beautiful lettuce that has it all, and which we feel is one of the best lettuces in the world. Will

---

stay fresh and tasty at marketable size for about three weeks even in hot weather without going to seed. Its heirloom flavor is epicurean.

Russian Red Kale: Considered to be both the hardiest and most delicate kale. A gourmet item. Very beautiful red oak–type leaves.

Good King Henry Greens for Salad: This rare plant, also known as Mercury and Lincolnshire Spinach, has fleshy long-stalked, arrow-shaped leaves. The roots some like better than asparagus. Delicious flower clusters. Will grow anywhere, but responds best to good cultivation. Potherb cooked and eaten much like spinach, also used in salads. Rich in vitamins A & C, calcium.

Red Drumhead Cabbage: Fine, sweet flavor—probably the best of all red cabbages.

Mayo Amaranth: A rare, Mexican grain/leaf variety from Jim Bowman of Louisiana (who saved the Fote Te variety). He claims it's the best leaf he has ever tasted.

Orach: One of the oldest cultivated vegetables in the world. Its leaves make an excellent spinach. Grows straight up on 2'–3' stalks, so good for compact gardens.

FRUIT

Baron Solemacher Strawberry: This is the Alpine Strawberry which is perennial and nonlayering. It has fantastic taste. Reproduces itself exactly from seed and is most vigorous and productive when grown from seed. With encouragement, can yield almost as abundantly in late summer as in spring.

Northern Arizona Melon: Anthony Shelley sent us seeds of this gem of a melon. "Growing up in Northern Arizona a spectacular melon grew. This melon can be much larger than a cantaloupe variety. The skin turns yellow when ripe with cantaloupe-orange flesh. The sweetness is better than any cantaloupe variety offered. This melon . . . was brought out West with the pioneers . . . who knows from there, perhaps Japan."

Moon and Stars Watermelon: One hundred days' growth—legendary cultivars rediscovered by Kent Whealy of the Seed Savers Exchange.

Large, oval fruits (20–40 pounds) have thin, brittle skins splashed with irregular, bright yellow shapes, reminiscent of moon and stars.

VEGETABLES

Offenham Parsnip: An early heirloom variety adapted to a wide variety of soil conditions, but especially prized for its ability to grow on thin, shallow soils. Half-long roots with broad, thick shoulders. The flesh is sweet, tender and has a fine flavor and quality. Good freezer. Very heavy yielding. Saved by backyard gardener Edward Marshall.

Amish Heirloom Sugar Snap Pea: Nearly stringless peas on vine 4"–6" tall. Prolific yield of moderately sweet peas in beautiful translucent pods. No diseases in five years of testing by our grower. Seed Savers Exchange variety via Betty Lamb via the Scatterseed Project. "Collected from an Amish man in Lancaster County, PA. . . . "

Brandywine Tomato: Heirloom pink Amish variety that dates back to 1885, and is one of the all-time finest flavored tomatoes. Strong flavor really brandylike in its intensity and richness. Vigorous potato-leafed vines that do well under most garden conditions.

Black Aztec Corn: A very ancient variety grown by the Aztecs 2,000 years ago. Still very competitive, with medium-sized white ears that are good for eating when in early maturity. Dried they become jet black, and are one of the finest blue flours and meals. Vigorous grower. Drought tolerant.

Canadian Orchard Baby Corn: From the Heritage Seed Program in Canada. A yellow sweet corn with fine flavor which matures as early as any hybrid! Small 3'–5' plants each produce 1–3 small 4"–6" ears which have full, juicy kernels and a fine, sweet taste.

Jimmy Nardello's Sweet Italian Frying Pepper: Heavy producer of long 6"–8", narrow .75"–1", thin-walled fruits colored green to bright red. Fruits mild and very sweet for a pepper, excellent taste. Great for frying, eating raw.

FINDING VARIETY IN YOUR COMMUNITY

When most of us think of apples we think of the familiar McIntosh, Delicious, Empire, and possibly Ida Reds. Unfortunately, there are not usually more than six varieties found in supermarkets. What a tragedy this is! Henry David Thoreau, in his 1862 essay "Wild Apples," wrote:

> *The era of the Wild Apple will soon be past: it is a fruit which will probably become extinct in New England . . . [H]e who walks over these fields a century hence will not know the pleasure of knocking off wild apples. . . . Ah, poor man . . . there are many pleasures which he will not know.*

The Greenmarket porgram of the Council on the Environment of New York City provides lists of fruits and vegetables available in their community. An organization in your location may offer something similar. Call your local Department of Agriculture office to find out. A quick perusal of the Greenmarket list provides a fascinating introduction to the variety of apples found within two hundred miles of New York City. The season starts in August with Red Gravensteins, Jerseyreds, Lodi, Early McIntosh, Miltons, Molly's Delicious, Paulareds, and Twenty-ounces, followed by an equal number of interesting-sounding varieties harvested until mid-November. Some farms are experimenting with July apples—they are very tart but delicious—and can be found at some farmers' markets.

There are a lot of varieties of other fruits and vegetables too. Most grocery stores offer only a few types of squashes, for example: acorn, butternut, and zucchini. To give you an idea of how limited this offering is, the Native Seeds/SEARCH seed catalog lists the following kinds of squashes that are traditional crops in the southwestern United States and northern Mexico alone: Mayo Blusher, Elfrida, Hopi "Vatnga," Papalote Ranch Cushaw, Parral Cushaw, San Bernardo, Silver Edged, Tarahumara, Tohono O'odham "Ha:l," Veracruz Pepita, Mayo Kama, Pima Bajo, Rio Mayo Big Cheese, Rio Fuerte Mayo Arrote, Rio Fuerte Mayo Segualca, Segualca, Acoma Pumpkin, Hopi Pumpkin, Mt. Pima Calabaza "Vavuli," Tarahumara, and Tepehaun "I:ma." Native Seeds/SEARCH is a nonprofit seed conservation organization working to preserve the traditional crops and their wild relatives of the U.S. Southwest and northern Mexico.

When you choose a variety of foods for optimum health and to support sustainable farms, don't confuse variety with the exotic. *Exotic* means from faraway places. If you live in northern Maine and buy some fruit from the South Pacific, while it will add a sort of variety to your diet, it had to travel eight thousand miles to get to you, which cost a lot in energy. And more than likely, that particular variety of fruit, which could stand up to long-distance travel, has been favored at the expense of other local varieties that may be tastier or more nutritious. Scour your community for locally grown, seasonal varieties of food instead.

STEP 5: EATING LOW ON THE FOOD CHAIN

Charles Elton, a zoologist from Cambridge University, coined the term *food chain* in 1927 to describe the nutritional dependencies linking species. Besides the sun, the first and most important link in the food chain is plants and soil bacteria, without which life would not exist. The second main link is herbivorous animals; and the third, carnivorous predators such as hawks, mountain lions, and humans. Each successive link eats the lower and more vulnerable species in the sequence. A bird is higher on the food chain than a worm, for example, as is a fish than a fly, or a cow than grass. Generally, the smallest species are at the bottom of the food chain, while larger animals are at the top, although nature always provides plenty of exceptions to any rule. Interestingly, those high on the food chain are the most superfluous. It is ironic that the world would survive without carnivorous predators but not without plants and bacteria.

Humans can eat both high and low on the food chain and be adequately nourished. The vast majority of Americans choose to eat at the top of the food chain, eating a wide range of animal products such as beef, pork, chicken, fish, milk, cheese, and eggs. This meat-based diet has a profound impact on human health and on the environment at large.

HEALTH

Vegetarian Seventh-Day Adventists have 50 percent less cancer overall, and 97 percent less colon cancer, than the general meat-eating public. Studies from around the world report that the lower a human being eats on the food chain, the more protected he or she will be against heart disease, cancer, and diabetes. "Studies of vegetarians indicate that they often have lower mortality rates from several chronic degenerative diseases than do non-vegetarians," notes the American Dietetic Association. Researchers present two reasons for the lower incidence of disease in vegetarian diets: animal products are very high in fat, and they have no fiber.

A 1995 study by doctors who are members of the Physicians Committee for Responsible Medicine estimates that the medical costs associated with a meat diet are between $28.6 billion and $61.4 billion a year. High blood pressure, heart disease, diabetes, and cancer are a few of the illnesses they link to diets high in red meat and poultry.

FAT

CHEMICAL CONCENTRATION IN THE FAT OF ANIMAL PRODUCTS

Residues of persistent chemicals such as DDT, PCBs, dioxin, and many pesticides concentrate in animal fat. If you follow the life of PCB molecules, for example, as is eloquently done in the book *Our Stolen Future,* you watch PCBs accumulate in higher and higher concentrations the further up the food chain you go.

As PCBs work their way up the food chain, their concentrations in animal tissue can be magnified up to 25 million times. Microscopic organisms pick up persistent chemicals from sediments, a continuing source of contamination, and water and are consumed in large numbers by filter feeding tiny animals called zooplankton. Larger species like mysids then consume zooplankton, fish eat the mysids, and so on up the food web to the herring gull.

Whereas the phytoplankton may have a concentration of 250 parts per billion of PCBs, the herring gull has a concentration twenty-five million times that of the phytoplankton. Eagles living along the shores of lakes and oceans eat herring gulls, multiplying their PCB contamination by another twenty times, which may explain why so many of them have died out, the authors speculate. The EPA reports that 90 percent of human exposure to dioxin occurs from diet, and most is from animal products.

So what if we have such high concentrations of dioxin and PCBs in our fat? you might ask. The authors of *Our Stolen Future* hypothesize, from their observation of threatened wildlife around the world, that many of these chemicals, which are now found all over the earth (even in the far reaches of the Arctic), are linked to reproductive problems, cancers, and neurological disorders. Scientists including those at the prestigious U.S. National Academy of Sciences and the EPA are investigating the connection between endocrine and hormone disruption exhibited in wildlife as a result of contamination with chemicals, and how the same chemicals may manifest themselves in humans. These contaminants can be passed from mother to child through breast milk and by exposure while in the womb. Humans are at the top of the food chain.

A 1980 study done of the chlorinated pesticide DDT's contamination of mothers' breast milk found that 99 percent of meat eaters had significant levels of DDT, whereas only 8 percent of the vegetarian mothers' milk had significant levels of DDT. You can reduce your exposure by eating fewer animal products, and when you do eat them, eat low-fat varieties of dairy products, and trim off the fat and buy lean varieties of meat.

THE WRONG KIND OF FAT AND HEART DISEASE

Death rates from heart disease are lower in vegetarians than in carnivores. Animal products are a major source of saturated fat and cholesterol in the diet, both of which increase blood levels of total cholesterol and LDL cholesterol, and thus increase the risk for coronary heart disease, according to the FDA. The National Cholesterol Education Program recommends a diet with no more than 30 percent fat, of which no more than 10 percent comes from saturated fat. Saturated fat is found mainly in animal products, but also in coconuts and palm oils.

DIABETES

Vegetarians are less likely to acquire non–insulin-dependent diabetes mellitus. While no one knows for certain why this is, researchers speculate that vegetarians eat more complex carbohydrates and fiber, which helps to slow the release of insulin, resulting in a lower basal blood glucose level. Also, fewer vegetarians are obese, which is also a contributing factor.

CANCER

There is a correlation between meat-based diets and colon cancer. Researchers have isolated two hypotheses for why this is so: first, meat-based diets are high in fat, and second, they are low in fiber. Fiber affects cholesterol levels, taking cholesterol with it as it leaves the body, and also helps move food through the intestines more quickly. People whose diets are high in fiber tend to have a low incidence of colon cancer. The National Cancer Institute recommends eating twenty to thirty grams of fiber a day. Reaching this goal is hard to accomplish if a large part of one's diet consists of meat, since it does not have any fiber. Finally, because vegetarians eat fewer animal products, their exposure to carcinogenic pesticides stored in animal fat is reduced. It should be noted, however, that researchers have not yet proven any risk of cancer from pesticides stored in animal fat.

ENVIRONMENTAL COST OF AN ANIMAL-BASED DIET

Modern meat production involves intensive use of grain, water, energy, and grazing areas. Pork is the most resource intensive, followed by beef, then poultry, eggs, and dairy products. Almost half of the energy used in American agriculture goes into livestock production. Industrialized farms raise animals as if they were merchandise, and such mechanized farming systems need energy to maintain the enormous "barns" in which the animals are penned: the buildings need to be heated, cooled, and lighted and the animals need to be transported to slaughter, processed in assembly lines run by electricity, and finally refrigerated.

There are three times more livestock than human beings on the earth, and animals require land to live on and land for their feed to be grown on. Rain forests are being deforested to make grazing land, and land is losing its topsoil from being overgrazed.

Animal agriculture produces surprisingly large amounts of air and water pollution. Overcrowding on industrial meat farms causes massive sewage pollution of water. Methane—a gas produced by the decomposition of sewage (of which livestock contributes a large amount) and other organic compounds—contributes to global warming.

Cattle and other livestock consume 90 percent of the soy and 70 percent of the grain grown in the United States, and according to the USDA, livestock worldwide consumes half the world's total grain harvest. It is sobering to realize that the soy and grain harvest used for livestock could feed human beings from around the world who are starving, forty to sixty million of whom die each year. And the feed that the animals eat has usually been intensively sprayed with pesticides, further contributing to air and water pollution.

A startling fact is that much of the world's fish population is fed to livestock. According to Worldwatch Institute's *1995 State of the World,* "approximately a third of the marine fish catch goes to other uses [besides food for humans]—primarily animal feed for pets, livestock, and pond-raised fish." Yet Lester Brown of the Worldwatch Institute notes, "United Nations' estimates indicate that all 17 of the world's major fishing areas have either reached or exceeded their natural limits and that nine are in decline. . . . Growth in output of oceanic fisheries has come to a halt." Are fish becoming an endangered species just to support the world's meat-eating habits?

Supplies of another one of the earth's most precious resources—if not the most precious—groundwater, are dwindling around the world. Figures of how many gallons of water it takes to produce one pound of meat range from an average of 2,500 gallons to upward of 5,000 gallons for beef. It takes about 130 gallons of water to produce a pound of milk.

Clearly a reduction in the world's consumption of meat will be a step toward preserving the healthy ecology of the earth and her precious resources. Diets of food found lower on the food chain—

largely plant-based—take a significantly lower environmental toll. Besides the benefits to the environment at large, there will also be more food to go around.

Eating Less Meat

The Dietary Guidelines for Americans state that vegetarian diets are perfectly acceptable for meeting the Recommended Dietary Allowances (RDAs) for vitamins, minerals, and protein. It stresses that vegetarians should be sure to eat an adequate amount and variety of food to ensure in particular proper amounts of protein, iron, zinc, and B vitamins, components typically found in higher amounts in meat, poultry, and fish.

The transition to eating less meat can be a process that takes months, even years. Some people, of course, choose to become a vegetarian overnight, and can make the transition easily. The USDA's food pyramid recommends legumes, nuts, and eggs as adequate protein substitutes for meat. Milk, yogurt, and cheese are considered adequate protein sources as well. A common pitfall of early-stage vegetarianism, however, is to rely heavily on dairy products, especially cheese, for protein. The problem with this approach is that though eating cheese is fine in moderation, a diet relying heavily on cheese is high in fat and high enough on the food chain for the fat to be contaminated with pesticides, PCBs, and dioxin. Beans and tofu—tasty though maligned in the media—are ideal sources of protein.

Others prefer to make the transition to eating less meat more gradually, substituting vegetarian sources of protein two to three meals a week. If you are part of the latter group, you might want to consider following the recommendations of the Asian Food Pyramid, developed by Oldways Preservation & Exchange Trust, a group dedicated to promoting environmentally sustainable foods and agricultural systems. The Asian Food Pyramid recommends eating eggs and poultry weekly; fish or dairy daily (an optional choice); and other meat, such as beef, monthly. The Asian Food Pyramid recommends eating fruits, legumes, nuts and seeds, vegetables, and grains daily.

Choosing the Meat You Eat from Sustainable Farms

There is one very important reason sustainable farms raise animals for the health of their farms: manure. Farm families are never able to keep all the animal babies—calves, chicks, piglets, lambs—that are born to a farm. It would not be practical. But if the meat you choose to eat has been raised on such a farm, you are assured that there is a very good chance the animal you are eating was raised humanely and ethically, without antibiotics and other hormones, and that it has been fed wholesome food. For more about purchasing organic animal products, see step 1, earlier in this chapter.

Vegetarian Diets

There are 12.5 million vegetarians in the United States, and the number is growing all the time. A lacto-ovo vegetarian eats dairy products and eggs, a lacto-vegetarian eats dairy foods but no eggs, and a vegan eats no animal foods of any kind.

Special Note about Vegan Diets

In the new Dietary Guidelines for Americans, the USDA and the USDHHS advise that vegans must supplement their diets with an adequate source of B_{12} by taking supplements. The only source of vitamin B_{12} is animal products, although some claim fermented food is a source. The American Dietetic Association does not believe that spirulina, seaweed, tempeh, and other fermented foods are reliable sources of vitamin B_{12}. The other two nutrients of concern for vegans, especially for vegan children, is obtaining adequate amounts of vitamin D and calcium, both found in milk (vitamin D is added to milk by most dairies).

Protein

Vegetarian diets of the 1970s emphasized food combining as a way of receiving complete proteins. Protein is made up of amino acids, and since all plant foods except soy have incomplete amino acid profiles, one needs to combine foods such as grains and dairy products, for example, to obtain a complete protein, in each meal. It is now believed that you need to eat a variety of foods of different amino acid content over an entire day to fulfill your protein requirements, not in each meal. Eating a variety of foods from the six food groups of the USDA's food pyramid will provide you with all your amino acid requirements.

HIGH-NUTRIENT FOODS

Vegetarian diets can be diverse and delicious. Once the basics are understood it is very easy to implement a healthful vegetarian diet. Pay particular attention to eating foods rich in zinc, calcium, B_{12}, and iron. If you eat a varied diet you should be getting all the nutrients you need.

Nuts and seeds are high in the mineral zinc, as are beans and whole grains. Beans, nuts and seeds, seaweeds, whole grains, and some fruits are high in iron. B_{12} is considered to be available only in animal products and needs to be supplemented. Calcium is widely available in dairy products, tofu (if processed with calcium sulfate), and dark green leafy vegetables such as kale, mustard greens, and turnip greens. Vitamin D is manufactured by the body when a person is exposed to the sun. Light-skinned people need about fifteen minutes of sun exposure a day for adequate vitamin D synthesis; those with dark skins need twice that.

STEP 6: EATING WHOLE FOODS WITH ADEQUATE FIBER

An apple, or even a sugarcane stalk, is a whole food that is nutritionally complex. Transforming an apple into apple sauce refines it to a degree. Making an apple into apple juice refines it further. Filtering the apple juice refines it even more. As more and more components of the fruit are removed, the more refined it becomes, and the more refined the food, the more stripped it is of nutrients. Whole foods—including fruits, vegetables, unrefined grains, nuts, and seeds—are the most healthful foods we can eat because they contain complex carbohydrates, fiber, and a host of other nutrients.

A leading proponent of eating whole foods, Annemarie Colbin, author of *Food and Healing* and *The Book of Whole Meals,* uses the example of sugar to describe the process of refinement and its effects. "When we take a food like sugarcane, then draw out the juice, strip the fiber, then filter out more nutrients until it is refined to the point that it is 99 percent pure carbohydrate, we have a food that is not found in nature. When we put it in our bodies, it feels as if something is missing," she teaches. To illustrate the point, if we eat toast made from refined white flour in the morning, many of us may then spend the rest of the day overeating in search of the missing nutrients—the rest of the wheat kernel, as it were. Crucial nutrients necessary to health, and necessary to metabolism of the carbohydrate, are missing from the refined and fragmented food, and our bodies may crave them.

Whole Foods versus Refined Foods

Flours from grains are commonly "refined." This means that the bran and the germ—the most nutritious parts of the grain, and highest in fiber—have been taken out and the flour is no longer whole, nor nutritionally as healthful. Most pasta (except for 100 percent whole wheat), light-colored breads, baked goods, and desserts are made of "white" flour, a flour that has been stripped of some of its most valuable nutrients, such as the E, A, and B vitamins and fiber. In fact one-half cup of unbleached white flour has no fiber, whereas one-half cup of whole wheat flour has eight grams, a significant difference. "Enriched" flour has some of the nutrients added back in, but not all. Fiber, enzymes, and many vitamins and minerals are not returned. The comparison in nutritional value between refined and unrefined wheat flour is striking.

Eating whole grains is crucial to your health. Whole grains have been shown to reduce the risk of heart disease and cancer by providing essential nutrients like vitamin E and considerable amounts of fiber. The American Dietetic Association reports a significant correlation between high intake of whole grains and a reduction in many serious diseases including cancer and heart disease. Unfortunately, most of us do not come close to eating enough *whole* grains every day—in fact many are lucky if they have one serving of whole grains a week!

For more on whole grains, see chapter 4, "The Green Pantry."

FRUITS AND VEGETABLES

The National Cancer Institute recommends we each "strive for five" servings of fresh fruits and vegetables a day, since the complex carbohydrates and fiber they contain play a very beneficial role in protecting against cancer, heart disease, and common digestive ailments. Yet less than one-third of American adults met that recommendation in 1995, according to the USDA and the USDHHS.

If you spread five servings of fruits and vegetables out over three meals a day plus snacks, ensuring that even a child reaches the goal of five servings a day isn't so hard. If you eat a vegetable for lunch and dinner, and fruit at two meals and a snack, you'll be all set. If you are unable to have a vegetable for lunch, you can have a salad and a vegetable for dinner.

FIBER

Impressive health claims are made about high-fiber diets. Reportedly they may reduce incidences of colon and other cancers, lower cholesterol, reduce the rate of heart disease, and lower the blood sugar of diabetics. There are two kinds of fiber, soluble and insoluble, both of which are found in plant foods such as grains, nuts, and seeds, as well as fruits and vegetables, and both of which are necessary for good health. Insoluble fiber does not dissolve in water, such as the hull around grains. Soluble fiber, such as oat bran, becomes glutinous when in contact with water. Most foods contain both kinds of fiber.

A Harvard School of Public Health study of nearly forty-four thousand male health professionals found that those with diets highest in fiber had 35 percent fewer heart attacks than those who ate a low-fiber diet. Those with a high-fiber diet had the lowest risk of heart attack regardless of how much fat and cholesterol they ate.

Researchers speculate that a high-fiber diet reduces the risk of

Fiber Content of Foods

Food	Serving Size	Fiber (grams)
Barley, pearl	1 cup cooked	6
Buckwheat flour	1 cup flour	12
Cornmeal	1 cup	9
Millet	1 cup cooked	3
Oats	1 cup cooked	4
Rice, brown	1 cup cooked	4
Rice, brown	1 cup flour	7
Rye	1 cup flour	29
Wheat, whole	1 cup flour	14
Black beans	1 cup cooked	14
Black-eyed peas	1 cup cooked	12
Garbanzo beans	1 cup cooked	10
Great Northern beans	1 cup cooked	12
Kidney beans	1 cup cooked	12
Lentils	1 cup cooked	16
Mung beans	1 cup cooked	15
Navy beans	1 cup cooked	16
Peas	1 cup cooked	16
Pinto beans	1 cup cooked	15
Soybeans	1 cup cooked	10
Almonds	1 cup	15
Cashews	1 cup	4
Filberts	1 cup	9
Peanuts	1 cup	12
Pecans	1 cup halves	8
Pumpkin seeds	1 cup	22
Sunflower seeds	1 cup	15
Walnuts	1 cup	6
Artichoke	1 medium	6
Asparagus	1 cup	5
Beans, snap	1 cup cooked	4
Broccoli	1 cup cooked	5

Fiber Content of Foods (continued)

Food	Serving Size	Fiber (grams)
Brussels sprouts	1 cup cooked	6
Carrot	1 cup grated	4
Cauliflower	1 cup cooked	4
Corn	1 cup cooked	4
Eggplant	1 cup cooked	2
Kohlrabi	1 cup cooked	3
Okra	1 cup cooked	4
Parsnips	1 cup cooked	3
Peas, edible pods	1 cup	4
Potato	1 cooked	4
Pumpkin	1 cup	4
Rutabagas	1 cup cooked	4
Salsify	1 cup cooked	3
Spinach	1 cup raw	1
Squash		
yellow summer	1 cup cooked	4
zucchini	1 cup cooked	4
butternut	1 cup cooked	5
acorn	1 cup cooked	6
Sweet potato	1 cup cooked	8
Turnip	1 cup cooked	4
Apple, raw whole	1 medium	4
Apricots	2	2
Avocado	1 medium	8
Banana	1 medium	3
Blueberries	$\frac{1}{2}$ cup	2
Cantaloupe	$\frac{1}{2}$	2
Cherries	1 cup	3
Grapefruit	$\frac{1}{2}$ medium	2
Mango	1	4
Nectarine	1	2
Orange	1 medium	3
Papaya	$\frac{1}{2}$	3

Fiber Content of Foods (continued)

Food	Serving Size	Fiber (grams)
Peach	1 medium	2
Pear	1 medium	4
Plum	1 medium	1
Pomegranate	1	1
Raspberries	$\frac{1}{2}$ cup	3
Strawberries	$\frac{1}{2}$ cup	3
Tangerine	1 medium	2
Watermelon	1 cup	.5

(*Source: USDA figures.*)

heart disease because when fiber-rich carbohydrates are eaten, blood sugar levels do not get as high, which slows down the release of insulin. (The more refined the carbohydrate, the more quickly our body turns it into glucose, and insulin levels rise to handle the sugar rush.) High levels of insulin are a factor in heart disease and diabetes. Under a doctor's supervision, diabetics on high-fiber diets are actually able to reduce the amount of insulin they require. Lower insulin levels may also reduce cholesterol synthesis.

Dr. Denis Burkitt, a British physician, reported in the early 1970s that Africans had significantly fewer cases of colon cancer and other diseases such as diverticular disease and even varicose veins. He observed that the African diet was very high in fiber (sixty or more grams a day), and that in Africans the "gut transit time" and elimination of food waste was one-third that of meat-eating Europeans with a low-fiber diet. Among other benefits such as soft stools, the sped-up elimination of digested food on a high-fiber diet meant that poisons (intestinal bacteria) spent less time building up in the digestive track, thereby possibly preventing digestive ailments including constipation and ultimately colon cancer.

Dr. Burkitt's findings have been echoed by other scientists. A study at Memorial Sloan-Kettering Cancer Center found that a high-fiber diet could actually shrink precancerous growths of the colon. And researchers from around the world have found that people who eat a diet high in fiber have lower cancer rates overall.

How Much Fiber?

The recommended daily allowance for fiber is twenty to thirty grams. Some health practitioners recommend people eat as much as sixty grams a day. If you decide to increase your fiber intake, make sure you do it slowly and drink a lot of water. Too much fiber, too quickly, can cause constipation, just as can too little fiber.

STEP 7: AVOIDING PROCESSED FOOD

Avoiding Excessive Use of Sugar, Fat, and Salt

SUGAR

Next to "white" flour, the other most refined food in the American diet is sugar. The average American eats fourteen pounds of sweeteners a year.

"Pure" refined sugar made its debut in 1812, when a chemist invented a method of extracting the juice from the sugarcane and sugar beet, leaving the bulk and fiber behind. To make granulated sugar as we know it, the juice is then purified, filtered, concentrated, and boiled down until the syrup crystallizes. The resulting product is 99.9 percent sugar crystals, the ultimate in a refined carbohydrate. Refined sugars include white table sugar, turbinado (raw sugar that has been refined and cleaned), brown sugar (essentially the same as white sugar, with the addition of a small amount of molasses or caramel color), confectioners' sugar (sugar plus cornstarch), and corn syrup, produced from cornstarch. Glucose (dextrose), fructose, maltose, and lactose are also considered to be "sugars."

Contrary to common belief, sugar has not been found to cause either hyperactivity in children (this is still controversial) or diabetes. However, obesity can cause diabetes, and eating too many refined foods can cause obesity. Refined carbohydrates are full of empty calories, lacking nutritional value. The more refined the carbohydrate, the more quickly our bodies turn it into glucose, and insulin levels rise to handle the sugar rush. "Refined dietary sugars almost always turn into fats," warns Udo Erasmus, author of *Fats That Heal and Fats*

That Kill. "Our body stores excess glucose from times of feasting—as fat—for use in future times of famine," he explains.

Are any sweeteners more healthful than others? A common point many nutritionists make is that all carbohydrates made up of basic sugar units such as glucose or fructose act the same way in our bodies, so it doesn't matter if we eat sugar or rice syrup, the body will react the same way to both. But an important issue that is left out of this argument is that less-refined sugars such as black-strap molasses have retained much of their nutritive value, and it is precisely those values that may help the body handle the rise in glucose and the subsequent release of insulin. "Refined sugars need no digestion and are absorbed rapidly. They lack the co-factors, and our body cannot burn them properly," Udo Erasmus writes. However, too much sweetener of any kind isn't healthful, no matter how unrefined.

Refined sugars can actually leach nutrients from the body. High-fructose corn syrup is a popular alternative to sugar and is found in everything from soda to some brands of peanut butter. It has been determined, however, that this refined sweetener depletes the body's level of chromium, a mineral essential to the body's ability to use and digest sugar properly. When corn syrup is eaten in conjunction with sugar (soda and cake, for instance), chromium depletion is further aggravated. This can lead to an increase in triglycerides and blood cholesterol—increases that factor into our risk for diabetes and heart disease.

For a glossary of whole food sweeteners and fruit sweeteners, please see chapter 3.

FAT

Almost all health professionals recommend a low-fat diet. High-fat diets increase the risk of cancer and heart disease. Yet in the panic about high-fat diets, many lump all fat together as being bad. This is misleading. The American diet tends to be high in the wrong kinds of fat (animal products and tropical oils), and low in the right kind of fat (essential fatty acids such as the omega-3 oils). The FDA's dietary guidelines point out that some dietary fat is essential. Essential fatty acids supply energy and promote absorption of the fat-soluble vitamins A, D, E, and K. The FDA recommends a diet with less total fat, saturated fat, and cholesterol.

Cholesterol is only found in animal products, and saturated fat is primarily found in animal products. Current guidelines recommend obtaining less than 30 percent of calories from fat. Many health practitioners believe the number should be even lower, 10 or 20 percent. (Most Americans get 40 percent of their calories from fat.) The most important issue regarding fat intake, besides making strides toward having less than 30 percent of one's daily calories come from fat, is what kind of fats you consume.

Essential Fatty Acids: Omega-3 and Omega-6

Essential fatty acids are the two oil molecules that the body cannot make for itself. Crucial for life and well-being, these essential fatty acids are available in some foods. These two "essential" oils are omega-3 and omega-6. Omega-3 oils are found in pumpkin, canola, wheat germ, rice bran, flax, walnuts, and soy. Omega-6 oils are found in all vegetable oils, particularly safflower, sunflower, corn, and sesame oil. Another reason to eat whole grains is that the bran and germ contain essential fatty acids.

Dr. Sidney Baker, a leading pioneer in the field of environmental health, believes that "at present, there is an epidemic in our culture of a deficiency of the essential fatty acid supplied by the omega-3 oils, which are oils with a high content of alpha-linolenic acid." How could anyone in our society have a deficiency of fat? you might ask. Dr. Baker believes that the reason for this epidemic is the change in the methods of processing vegetable oils, which began around 1950, where essential fatty acids are actually removed from oils in the interest of preserving their shelf life. More saturated oils, such as corn, palm, peanut, safflower, and sunflower oils, are also preferred by manufacturers because their shelf life is longer. Baker concludes that "the trade-off for longer shelf life and the widespread distribution of vegetable oils has been that people have been susceptible to an imbalance of the substances contained in these oils that make for healthy, flexible cell membranes."

Symptoms of fatty acid deficiency include dry skin, lusterless hair, soft fingernails that break easily, and little raised "chicken" bumps on the back of the arms and sometimes the thighs. A recent study from the National Institute on Alcohol Abuse and Alcoholism links omega-3 deficiency and increase in depression and aggression.

A special note should be made about linseed oil. Food-grade linseed oil is now available in most health food stores in the country. You will—or should—find it in the refrigerator. Do not ever confuse food-grade linseed oil with the kind of linseed oil one typically finds in hardware stores and that is used for painting. Drying chemicals and other solvents have been added to those products.

Another reason to reduce overall fat intake is that fats and oils promote the production of free radicals. Free radicals are chemicals that occur in the body and attack cells and thereby contribute to diseases such as cancer and cardiovascular disease. Oxygen causes free radicals to develop in oils. However, oils rich in essential fatty acids and antioxidants such as vitamin E have been shown to neutralize free radicals and protect us from cell damage.

Saturated Fat

The Dietary Guidelines for Americans states that "saturated fat raises blood cholesterol more than any other forms of fat." Authoritative studies abound that link diets high in saturated fat and cholesterol with the risk of heart disease. All animal products contain saturated fat, whereas few vegetable oils do. (Tropical plants such as avocado, peanut, and coconut are the exceptions. They contain around 18 to 20 percent.) Canola is the oil with the lowest saturated fat concentration, at 6 percent.

Saturated fat, butter being a perfect example, is solid at room temperature. The higher the concentration of saturated fat in vegetable oils, the thicker the oil. Whereas the Dietary Guidelines recommend less than 30 percent of calories come from fat, they also recommend that only 10 percent of calories should be from saturated fat. Ways to reduce your intake of saturated fat include cutting back on meat and choosing low-fat or skim milk. Read labels carefully; many baked goods contain lard, beef tallow, or coconut oil.

Unsaturated Fats

Less stable than saturated fats, unsaturated fats remain liquid at room temperature. Unsaturated fats—or those with the lowest concentrations of saturated fats—include canola, safflower, and flaxseed.

Monounsaturated and Polyunsaturated Oils

Both monounsaturated and polyunsaturated oils are linked to reducing serum cholesterol. Some studies suggest that monounsaturated oils don't at the same time reduce HDLs (high-density lipoproteins), or "good" cholesterol, hence olive and canola oils' claim to fame. (Olive oil has 82 percent monounsaturates, canola has 60 percent.) Other unrefined oils relatively high in monounsaturated fats include almond, peanut, pistachio, pecan, canola, avocado, hazelnut, cashew, and macadamia oils.

Unrefined polyunsaturated oils are high in omega-6, and include safflower oil (79 percent polyunsaturated), sunflower oil (69 percent), corn oil (60 percent), and soy oil (50 percent).

Note: Make sure not to mistake trans-polyunsaturated (hydrogenated and partially hydrogenated) oils as acceptable oils, as they can interfere with the metabolism of essential fatty acids. For more on this, see below.

Superunsaturated Oils

Superunsaturated oils are an excellent choice because they are very high in omega-3. Flax oil is by far the highest source at 57 percent superunsaturated, followed by pumpkin seed (15 percent), canola (10 percent), soy (8 percent), and walnut oil (5 percent).

Hydrogenated/Partially Hydrogenated Oils/Trans-fatty Acids

In the rush to replace solid, spreadable butter, which is full of saturated fat and cholesterol, scientists came up with a process called hydrogenation. Hydrogenated and partially hydrogenated fats are made up of preferable unsaturated fats, but they are artificially hardened. Margarine is an example. Advertised as not containing cholesterol or saturated fat, hydrogenated oils seemed the answer for those concerned about heart disease. Trans-fatty acids are derived primarily from hydrogenated and partially hydrogenated oils. Although there are many concerns about the havoc trans-fatty acids may play in the body, including atherosclerosis and cancer, one concern is that if too many trans-fatty acids are ingested, they interfere with essential fatty acid function. Given that many Americans may be borderline deficient in omega-3 oils to begin with, interference in their function is not recommended for optimum health!

The body doesn't appear to know quite what to do with solid vegetable oils, and in 1990 Dutch researchers concluded that artificially hydrogenated oils and trans-fat may in fact raise serum cholesterol levels almost as much as saturated fats do.

Read labels very carefully to avoid hydrogenated, partially hydrogenated, or trans-fatty acids. They are found in everything from mayonnaise to cookies to breads.

Artificial Fat Substitute Olestra

A new, synthetic fat substitute named olestra has recently been approved by the FDA. Olestra adds no fat or even calories to foods such as potato chips, crackers, and other snacks. Sound like a miracle food? Unfortunately there is a hitch. The FDA is requiring that a warning label be placed on all food products that contain olestra. It reads, "This product contains Olestra. Olestra may cause abdominal cramping and loose stools. Olestra inhibits the absorption of some vitamins and other nutrients. Vitamins A, D, E, and K have been added."

What this label doesn't make clear is that olestra can not only inhibit the absorption of some vitamins and other nutrients found in the food processed with olestra, but can take all those nutrients it finds in the intestines, including carotenoids, with it as well. Carotenoids, found in fruits and vegetables, are associated with lower cancer risk. If your child eats an apple while she nibbles on some olestra potato chips, she may well lose the nutritional benefits of the apple! While vitamins A, D, E, and K have been added to the olestra-based snacks, experts in public health report that nobody knows exactly which nutrients are being depleted, or how much to replace of the ones they do know are being lost. A whole foods diet is geared to provide one's body, or one's family's bodies, with an optimum number of nutrients. Olestra does not belong in a whole foods diet.

Note: See chapter 3 for how to buy and identify unrefined oils high in essential fatty acids.

SODIUM AND SALT

There is a firmly associated relationship between sodium and high blood pressure (hypertension). Consequences of high blood pressure include heart and kidney disease and strokes. Salt (a combination of sodium and chlorine) is in the salt shaker on most tables in America, but the highest quantities are found in processed and prepared foods. High intakes of salt may also increase the amount of excreted calcium.

The average American consumes about three teaspoons of salt a day. Those of us who eat a lot of convenience, processed, and prepackaged foods are probably getting much more salt than we ever imagined. The sodium content is much higher in canned foods than in fresh food. Be particularly wary of canned soups, baked goods, dairy products such as cheese, and pickles and other fermented foods. One can of soup can have 750 milligrams of salt, for example, two slices of bread 250 milligrams, and one-half cup of flavored rice mix 250 to 400 milligrams. Watch out for ham, which can have over 1,000 milligrams of sodium in just three ounces, or vegetables frozen or canned with a sauce, which can contain almost 500 milligrams for just one-half cup.

The National Academy of Sciences Recommended Daily Allowance for minimum intake of sodium is only 500 milligrams a day for an adult—less than $\frac{1}{4}$ teaspoon! To determine how much salt you actually add to foods, the USDA recommends you take the shaker test. Simply cover your dinner plate with wax paper or foil. Salt as you would normally, and then collect the salt and measure it.

Look for "low-sodium" (140 milligrams or less per serving), "very low sodium" (35 milligrams or less), or "sodium free" (less than 5 milligrams) labels when you buy packaged foods in particular, and read the label. Try to reduce your consumption of dill pickles, bouillon, olives, soy sauce, and packaged dinners. Experiment with different kinds of spices such as thyme, curry, marjoram, and basil, instead of using salt for flavor.

Avoiding Possibly Harmful Chemicals and Additives

The average American eats 150 pounds of additives a year, much of which is sugar and salt, but by no means all. Three thousand additives are intentionally used in processed foods. Unintentional additives contribute many thousand pounds more. What are these additives doing to us?

Many of the additives are perfectly harmless, but some may be a concern for health. Additives don't belong in a whole foods diet. Some additives are especially bad for children. The Feingold Association of America has worked tirelessly in its belief that children are more sensitive to food additives, just as they are to chemicals, and that testing food additives for their cancer-causing properties does not address issues of neurotoxicity and the cause of behavioral disturbances.

There is a significant increase in diagnoses of childhood attention deficit disorder (ADD). Nationally the estimates are that between 3 and 10 percent of children have ADD; the Baltimore County school system medicates one in every seventeen children for the illness. The Feingold Association prescribes a diet free of many chemical additives based on phenol or that are considered neurotoxic, as well as natural salicylates. Many studies show that this more holistic approach to ADD is often a very successful way of controlling the illness. Artificial colors, artificial flavors, BHA (butylated hydroxyanisole), BHT (butylated hydroxytoluene), and TBHQ (tertiary butylhydroquinone) are avoided on the Feingold Diet, and these additives and a few others are on our list of additives of particular concern as well.

ADDITIVES OF PARTICULAR CONCERN

Artificial Sweeteners

Artificial sweeteners include aspartame (brands NutraSweet and Equal) and saccharin. They have no nutritive value and have never been shown to help people successfully lose weight.

The concept of sweetening without adding calories has obvious advantages, but saccharin has been linked to bladder cancer, and the use of aspartame may cause multiple health problems. In the body, aspartame is broken down into two amino acids and methanol. Amino acids are naturally occurring compounds that are used in the human body to synthesize proteins. Many researchers use the fact that amino acids are "natural" to support their view that aspartame is safe.

However, the consumption of naturally occurring amino acids can cause ill health when the amino acid balance in the body is upset. The two amino acids in aspartame, phenylalanine and aspartic acid, influence levels of neurotransmitters in the body. Neurotransmitters are molecules in the brain that affect mood and behavior. When neurotransmitters are out of balance, as they can be in a person who consumes aspartame, then adverse reactions can occur. Some people are particularly sensitive to aspartame, reporting effects such as headaches, blurred vision, dizziness, confusion, memory loss, irritability, and anxiety. Pregnant women are advised to avoid products containing aspartame altogether because one out of twenty thousand babies is born without the ability to metabolize phenylalanine.

For a glossary of whole food sweeteners and fruit sweeteners, please see chapter 3.

Sulfites, Sulfur Dioxide Gas

Sulfiting agents can cause death from anaphylactic shock in highly sensitive individuals. One million Americans are estimated to be sensitive to sulfites and can have mild to deadly reactions to them. Most sulfite-sensitive people are asthmatics. A typical reaction of those sensitive is difficulty breathing within a number of minutes of eating food containing sulfites. Sulfites are most commonly used to retain color in products such as fruits and vegetables.

Sulfiting agents are in a surprising number of products, including chili, almost all vinegars, dried fruit, potatoes, wine, shrimp, and so-called children's fruit snacks. Sulfiting agents can also be found in some very unexpected places: relishes, horseradish, sugar derived from sugar beets (including brown, white, and confectioners'), and some baked goods.

There are six sulfites, and the FDA has ranked them as Generally Regarded as Safe (GRAS): sulfur dioxide, sodium sulfite, sodium and potassium bisulfite, and sodium and potassium metabisulfite. Because it is agreed that sulfites can destroy vitamin B_1, they are not allowed to be used on meat or on other recognized sources of that vitamin.

Monosodium Glutamate (MSG)

MSG is often found in Chinese food, so those who are sensitive to MSG have symptoms that have been dubbed the Chinese Restaurant syndrome. Sensitivity symptoms include headaches; difficulty breathing; tingling in the hands, arms, and neck; heart palpitations; and feelings of numbness. MSG can be a serious threat to some asthmatics.

MSG is a sodium salt of glutamic acid, an amino acid, and by FDA definition, naturally occurring. However, as with aspartame, when amino acids are thrown out of balance with one another, serious consequences can result for some people. Some animal studies have raised concern. For example, infant mice fed large amounts of MSG had serious damage to their hypothalamus, and the same result has been seen in monkeys.

A food can be billed as having "natural flavors" and still contain MSG. Watch out for the following on ingredient labels: glutamate, monosodium glutamate, monopotassium glutamate, glutamic acid, calcium caseinate, sodium caseinate, gelatin, textured protein, hydrolyzed protein, yeast extract, yeast food, autolyzed yeast, and yeast nutrient, according to the Truth in Labeling Campaign. For other of the many, many label "descriptors" that often contain MSG or can create MSG during processing, including such items as malt extract and pectin, contact the Truth in Labeling Campaign in Darien, Illinois.

Sodium Nitrite and Sodium Nitrate

Sodium nitrate is used to help meat retain its color and as a meat preservative. It is commonly found in many luncheon meats. Sodium nitrate alone is considered harmless, but it combines in the body with saliva and bacteria to become nitrite, which in turn is converted by the body into nitrosamines, which are powerful carcinogens. As a result, nitrites are considered to be directly linked to cancer.

Vitamins C and E reportedly help inhibit the development of nitrosamines. While avoidance of meats containing sodium nitrate is the best course, whenever you eat meats that have nitrates in them, eat a pear or orange for vitamin C as well.

Artificial Food Coloring

Many artificial food dyes have been taken off the market because they have been found to be toxic or carcinogenic. Food dyes serve no useful purpose whatsoever and can often be used to deceive or lure consumers. At the moment there are only seven dyes on the market: Red No. 3, Red No. 40, Yellow No. 5, Yellow No. 6, Blue No. 1, Blue No. 2, and Green No. 3.

The FDA has estimated that between forty-seven thousand and ninety-four thousand Americans are sensitive to Yellow No. 5. It can cause asthma, hives, headache, and is linked to behavioral changes. In a double-blind study reported in the *Journal of Pediatrics,* children were tested to see if Yellow No. 5 could trigger behavioral reactions. The study clearly demonstrated a relation between the ingestion of Yellow No. 5 and behavioral changes in children who are allergic to it.

BHT and BHA

BHT (butylated hydroxytoluene) and BHA (butylated hydrox-yanisole) are commonly used as preservatives in some foods such as cereals and crackers to reduce rancidity. BHA is listed as a possible carcinogen with the World Health Organization and is considered an endocrine disrupter.

BHT is sometimes added to packaging cardboard. BHT may be toxic to the kidneys according to researchers at Michigan State University. It may also have a deleterious effect on those who take steroid hormones and oral contraceptives. BHT is prohibited in England.

If BHT and BHA are added to an ingredient used in a processed food, they need not be specifically listed. To avoid BHT and BHA you need to avoid processed foods.

Bioengineered Foods

Genetically engineered plants are modified by modern genetic techniques, such as recombinant DNA, which allow researchers to manipulate genetic material in ways not possible with traditional selective breeding. For example, researchers can transfer genetic material from one species to another, such as from animals to plants. As of the end of 1994, the U.S. Department of Agriculture had approved more than 1,100 field trials of genetically engineered crops. Close to market are potatoes, corn, soybeans, squash, and cotton (some grown for cottonseed oil).

A major health concern about genetic engineering is that the new products may cause susceptible individuals to become allergic to foods they previously could safely consume. Bioengineered food is not currently labeled.

The *New England Journal of Medicine* reports that eight out of nine people sensitive to Brazil nuts had allergic skin reactions to soybeans that had Brazil nut genes spliced into them. Though the soybean in question was removed from the market, other products that have been produced by transferring characteristics from one organism to another will continue to be placed on the market.

A number of analysts believe that there should be special requirements to ensure the safety of bioengineered foods, but the FDA is not requiring any.

Unless the FDA changes its labeling policy, the only way you can knowingly avoid bioengineered foods is to stick to certified organic foods—something that may be particularly important for people with serious food allergies. For more on buying organic, see step 1 of this chapter.

BOVINE GROWTH HORMONE rBGH (rBST)

If 10 percent of the dairy cows in America—the number treated with rBST—were injected with a dye that produced blue milk, it would be hard to find dairy products made from white milk because the milk from many dairies is blended together at processing plants. We would see blue—or at least light blue—milk products in every refrigerator and cupboard in America because it would appear in our infant formulas, cheese, cottage cheese, yogurt, butter, medications, crackers, processed foods, and school lunches. If blue milk proved to be unsafe for humans, the health of virtually all Americans would be jeopardized.

Roughly 10 percent of cows in America are now being injected with a bioengineered bovine growth hormone to boost milk production (known as rBGH or rBST). Milk from rBST-treated cows is one of the first products of bioengineering the FDA has approved to enter our food supply. Yet numerous concerns have been raised by scientists about the safety of rBST.

Because rBST is a genetically engineered hormone it does not exist in nature. It has eight more amino acid residues than the natural bovine growth hormone. The FDA acknowledges that synthetic milk hormones "are about 0.5 to 3 percent different in molecular structure" from natural milk hormones.

The FDA warning for farmers on the rBST label reads: "Use of Posilac [the brand name of Monsanto's rBST] is associated with increased frequency of medication in cows for mastitis and other health problems." Other illnesses in the cows include heat intolerance, multiple complications of the reproductive system, disorders of the foot, and significant weight loss.

Antibiotics are used to treat mastitis, and because antibiotics used on cows ends up in the milk, the increased use on cows is a significant issue for the consumer. Resistance to antibiotics is of increasing and recognized concern as a major threat to successfully treating bacteria-based diseases in humans, such as tuberculosis and ear infections.

The rBST stimulates the cow's liver to produce another protein hormone—insulinlike growth factor (IGF–1). IGF-1 can be greatly increased in milk from rBST-treated cows. *If* absorbed by humans, increased IGF-1 is of serious health significance. In the coming years, this is the issue to keep most alert to concerning rBST and health. One concern is that IGF-1 helps to promote cell division. "A cell division factor like IGF-1 is termed a mitogen. And, IGF-1 in higher amounts is associated with colon tumors and breast tumor tissues," testified Dr. William von Meyer, a geneticist, at a hearing of the Food Advisory Panel of the FDA.

Humans don't have receptor sites for cow growth hormones of any sort, making the hormone inactive when ingested orally. However, the milk is changed by the indirect effects of rBST, such as the increase of IGF-1 and antibiotic residues mentioned above, raising serious health concerns. Besides these problems there can be an increase in the somatic cell count found in milk because of mastitis. Finally, the increase in illness in cows, and the discomfort of carrying so much more milk, is of humanitarian concern.

Because milk products from cows that have been treated with rBST are not labeled, it takes a special effort to find milk from untreated cows. Whenever possible buy certified organic dairy products, which are not derived from rBST-treated cows.

BIOTECHNOLOGY AND THE ENVIRONMENT

Ecologists warn that ecosystems can be threatened because agricultural uses of biotechnology aren't easily contained. One potentially devastating example from California, as reported in *Science News* (no. 127, 1985) and *Science* (no. 229, 1985), is a bioengineered version of bacteria found on plants. The natural bacteria are not ice resistant, while the bioengineered ones are. According to the experts, however, natural bacteria found on plants combine with soil and dirt, and are then blown into the atmosphere, where water collects around the particles and freezes. This process is crucial for the formation of rain. If the bioengineered bacteria blown into the atmosphere won't freeze, the result could be less rain.

Less rain? Clearly biotechnology is an industry rife with unknowns. There are many public concerns about agricultural biotechnology that need to be addressed. At present, government agencies do not appear equipped to adequately evaluate the profound social, economic, and ecological ramifications of biotechnology. We need to develop a public dialogue for concerns to be aired, to make certain that as a society, we make wise and carefully researched choices.

IRRADIATED FOODS

Food that is irradiated has been treated with
gamma radiation (X rays). Radiation is used
to kill microorganisms in food. It is used on
spices and produce to kill mold and bacteria,
on poultry to kill salmonella, and on pork to
kill trichina. The FDA may approve the irradiation of red meat soon.

*Radura symbol marks
irradiated food.*

The FDA has approved radiation doses for spices, produce,
pork, and poultry that is millions of times more intense than that
allowed in dental X rays. Whereas irradiation can kill microorganisms, it also creates "unique radiolytic products," the safety of
which has not been proved or disproved.

Irradiation also reduces the nutrient content of food. Some irradiated foods, such as pears, apples, and citrus fruits, actually spoil faster
after irradiation, so one wonders what the point of irradiation is.

A very good reason to avoid irradiated foods is to protest the
increase of radioactive material in our environment.

STEP 8: REDUCING PACKAGING FOR PUBLIC HEALTH AND THE ENVIRONMENT

Per person, Americans generate 4.4 pounds of municipal solid
waste a day. Packaging accounts for fully one-third of this. The EPA
estimates that by the year 2000 the amount of plastics we throw
away will increase by 50 percent. As it is, plastics take up 32 percent of landfills by volume. By weight, paper and paperboard take
up 30.2 percent, plastics 8 percent, glass 2.2 percent, and aluminum 2.4 percent.

Less than one percent of plastics manufactured in America are
currently recycled, according to the EPA. Thirty-four percent of paper
and paperboard is recycled; 20 percent of glass and 30 percent of metals are recycled. Of the total municipal solid waste stream, 80 percent
is landfilled, 10 percent is incinerated, and 10 percent recycled.

Five of the top six chemicals whose production generates the
most hazardous waste, as ranked by the EPA, are used in the plas-

tics industry. Dioxin and three hundred other organochlorines have been identified in the effluent from the pulp-bleaching process in paper mills.

The use of chlorine to bleach pulp and paper has been identified as a major source of dioxin in the environment. The production of plastic accounts for the single largest use of chlorine. Packaging accounts for 30 percent of the plastic manufactured, and 50 percent of U.S. paper. Our overuse of these packaging materials has grave and widespread consequences.

CHLORINE AND DIOXIN

Chlorine is a chemical element naturally found in ocean water and our bodies in the form of the chemical compound called sodium chloride, commonly known as table salt. Many synthetic chemical compounds that contain chlorine are linked to myriad health and environmental problems, including cancer; damage to the reproductive, developmental, endocrine, and immune systems; and depletion of the ozone layer.

These worrisome chemicals may be deliberately synthesized—for use as solvents or to make plastics, for example—or they may be accidental by-products or contaminants that result when chlorine is used. For example, disinfecting drinking water with chlorine results in by-products suspected of causing cancer. And the infamous dioxins and related compounds can form both during the manufacture of synthetic chlorinated chemicals and during their disposal in incinerators.

According to the EPA's most recent assessment (1994), *any* amount of dioxins causes some degree of harm. Dioxin causes cancer at lower doses than any other carcinogen, and it is also an endocrine disrupter. The EPA estimates that 31 percent of known emissions of dioxin come from municipal waste incineration. (*Note:* these emissions do not reflect emissions of the pulp, paper, or chemical industries.)

Not all plastic contains chlorine (thus, not all plastics produce dioxin in their incineration). Polyvinyl chloride plastic no. 3 (PVC) is the worst offender. Thirty-four percent of the global chlorine production is used to make PVC, according to Greenpeace. Most vinyls can't be recycled at all, and dioxins have been produced even in recycling

PVC products. The Swedish Ecocycle Commission stated in 1994, according to Greenpeace, that "recycling PVC cannot be recommended with today's technology. In the Commission's opinion it is not advisable to initiate the collection of PVC products on a large scale before the possible environmental impacts of recycling PVC are known." There is a direct correlation between how much PVC is being burned in an incinerator and how much dioxin the incinerator releases.

Dioxin and other chemicals including plastics are now considered to disrupt the endocrine system of wildlife and possibly humans. The chemicals may be responsible at least in part for the dramatic decline in sperm counts and increasing rates of breast, testicular, and prostate cancers, endometriosis, and some abnormalities present at birth, such as undescended testicles.

Plastics also contribute heavy metals to the waste stream, including lead and cadmium, as these metals are used in the manufacture of some plastics. The EPA estimates that 28 percent of all cadmium and 2 percent of all lead in municipal solid waste can be traced to plastics. Heavy metals may leach out of landfills and are also components of incinerator ash, causing a threat to those downwind.

Packaging and Wildlife

Most of us by now have heard the stories of marine animals such as seals entangled in plastic. Plastic is the major source of all the garbage found in harbors and on beaches. Some of it comes from garbage barges, some from sewage, and some from careless human littering. The EPA reports that entanglements and ingestion of plastic by marine animals affects seabirds, seals, whales, turtles, fish, and crustaceans. Birds and turtles are particularly vulnerable because they mistake plastic items for food. The Office of Technology Assessment concluded that plastic pollution is a greater threat to marine wildlife than pesticides, oil spills, and water contamination.

Discharges into the waterways from the manufacturing of plastic and paper add a high burden of toxic chemicals to aquatic life. Air pollution from the same manufacturing plants can cause problems too. As just one example, paper mills release chloroform into the air, which is considered a carcinogen in animals.

Toxic Chemicals Can Migrate to Your Food from Packaging

Dioxin in paper and chemicals in plastics can migrate into food. For example, everyone knows the taste of plastic found in plastic-bottled water that has been left in the sun. One should go to extremes to eliminate the circumstances that can cause such migrations of chemicals into food because, as discussed above, some of the materials used in packaging are endocrine disrupters. The following guidelines should help give you ideas of how to avoid food contamination from packaging.

Guidelines for Reducing Food Contamination from Packaging

* Plastic tends to migrate into fatty foods, especially hot fatty foods. Don't leave cheese wrapped in its plastic wrapper sitting in the sun! Cool leftovers before placing in plastic storage containers.

* Plastic wrap should never come into direct contact with fatty food in the microwave. It is also important not to use leftover margarine or yogurt tubs in the microwave. Use ceramic or glass cookware instead.

* Microwavable packages should be avoided. Polyethylene terephthalate (PET) migrates from the packaging into the food, as do the adhesive components (and their degraded products) of the package.

* A 1988 FDA study of microwavable packaging components, called heat susceptors, showed that low levels of the carcinogen benzene could migrate into food when heated.

* Skip the boil-in-a-plastic-bag foods, as well as *sous vide* foods—foods that are vacuum packed.

* When you can, replace plastic cups and other eating utensils that come into contact with hot fatty foods with glass or metal. For example, instead of buying a plastic thermos, consider a metal one.

* As much as possible, avoid food, water, and other beverages

sold in plastic containers and bottles. For example, try to buy water from distributors who can deliver large glass jugs in convenient dispensers.

* Package components can migrate into wet food, especially if the food contains alcohol, acid, or fat.

* Use substitutes for bleached paper products that can come in contact with food, such as gold coffee filters and glass bottles.

* Avoid packaging with antioxidant preservatives such as BHT, an additive with a questionable safety record.

* Avoid buying imported food in cans sealed by soldering; the soldering may contain lead. In 1991, American manufacturers agreed to stop packaging food in cans soldered with lead. However, food that has been canned and sealed with lead solder is still imported to the United States. Lead solder that is used to seal cans can leach into the food—especially acidic foods such as tomato sauces and food packaged with vinegar or lemon juice, such as canned artichoke hearts. Lead-soldered cans are bumpy feeling under the seam, as opposed to seamless or welded cans.

* Many cans have plastic coatings that line the inside of the can out of concern that the metal might contaminate the food. Eighty-five percent of the cans sold in the United States have such linings, and the plastic coating leaches substances into the food, which can disrupt the hormonal system, according to *Our Stolen Future*. When you buy the cans there is no way to tell which cans are lined with plastic and which aren't.

REUSING VIRGIN RESOURCES: RECYCLING

While the manufacturing of packaging has a profound environmental effect, not recycling the packaging once it has been made, and throwing it instead into the trash, makes the drain on virgin resources even more intense. For example, only 5 percent as much energy is required to produce a sheet of aluminum from recycled materials as is required to produce the original sheet from raw materials. The more aluminum that is recycled, the less bauxite ore needs to be mined from the earth. The more plastic that is recycled, the less dioxin will be released in incinerators. See chapter 3 for helpful ways to reduce your packaging consumption to begin with, and chapter 6 for recycling tips.

3

The New Foragers:
New Ways to Shop
and Acquire Whole Food

No matter where you live in the country, there are ways to find whole, unprocessed, and locally grown organic food. In fact, whole food is so flavorful and appealing, it is increasingly in demand and available. You may have to become something of a modern forager to find a steady and abundant supply, because while unprocessed and organic products are increasingly available, they can't be called mainstream.

There is at least one item in every food category found in supermarkets that has few additives and is minimally processed. A more plentiful supply of organic foods—particularly high-quality fruits and vegetables—is found in health food stores, natural food stores, green supermarkets, food co-ops, mail-order catalogs, farmers' markets, and local farms, to name a few. A typical health food store offers, on average, a hundred organically grown items in their produce department. Though 42 percent of mainstream supermarkets sell organically grown produce, they carry on average twelve items, according to the Food Marketing Institute.

A successful and common combination of approaches to acquiring fresh, whole food is to visit a supermarket or health food store once a week, order from a food co-op once a month, and find a source of local organic produce. Finding the latter can be the biggest challenge, but this chapter offers you a large number of ideas to get you started. Eventually, your appreciation of the flavor of local, organic fresh food will be all the motivation you will need to make the extra effort to find it.

CONVENTIONAL STORES

SUPERMARKETS

A big shift has taken place in mainstream supermarkets. In 1992 only 12 percent of senior supermarket managers felt that offering "natural" products was important, but in 1996, just four years later, the number has catapulted up to 51 percent, according to the Food Marketing Institute. This enormous increase in interest in offering natural products is very good news for us (even if it is unclear what they mean by *natural*). It appears we don't need to look far to find a sympathetic ear at our supermarkets, to ask for an increase in the amount of organic food offered. The more often we make requests for specific types of whole food, the more quickly change will happen.

One important caveat about shopping in supermarkets: you need to read ingredients labels to find foods for a green diet. But the effort is worth it because by doing so you will be able to meet many of the goals outlined in chapter 2. If you read carefully you will be able to find minimally processed brands that may not be organic and locally grown but will at least have few additives and be made of whole food.

GREEN SUPERMARKETS

The new green supermarkets—stores that make a business of offering a larger selection of whole food that is often organic—are doing a booming business. Fresh Fields, Alfalfas, Wild Oats, and Bread and Circus are examples of green supermarkets.

Green supermarkets have everything found in a normal supermarket—bakery, produce, dry goods, deli, meats—but with a difference: much is organic, and you are likely to find a greater percentage of whole and unprocessed foods than in a conventional supermarket. To get a better idea, imagine your favorite health food store in a building the size of most supermarkets, and then add unexpected bonuses such as a delicatessen with focaccia and pesto; and a bakery baking bread, cakes, and cookies with only organically grown whole grains and naturally colored frostings free of refined sugar. Add a wing of the store for natural meats, and another with mostly organic produce. You can even squeeze your own fruit juices on the premises, and buy nuts and seeds in bulk. They even offer green cleaning products!

To find green supermarkets, however, you need to live near a big city or very large town. For those of us who don't, local health food stores are the next best option.

HEALTH FOOD STORES

The food found in health food stores rarely contains additives (see chapter 2). The food is often whole and organic, but because it is found in a health food store (or green supermarket, for that matter) does not guarantee that it is organic or made of whole foods. In fact, many of the bakery items and pasta are made of refined wheat flour. You still need to read all labels. That being said, however, health food stores are sources of some wonderful food. The stores are excellent sources of soy products such as tofu; organic dairy including yogurt and cheese; eggs from free-range hens; locally grown organic produce and meats; whole grain cereals; Mexican food wrappers such as tortillas; and whole food snacks, including candy without food dyes, for special occasions. As with green supermarkets, health food stores tend to stock the greenest cleaning products available. As a general rule, the smaller the health food store, the more it will tend to carry primarily snacks and vitamins.

HOW THE GOVERNMENT HELPS: FOOD LABELS

If you shop in conventional stores and want to buy whole food, the best advice is to read ingredients labels for every food product you buy, as only that label will tell you the truth about the food you are buying. If the product has unappealing ingredients, pass it by and look at labels of like products until you find one that is a good choice. With very few exceptions we have found that there is a whole foods choice for every food product category.

The FDA is responsible for assuring that food sold in the United States is "safe, wholesome and appropriately labeled." The Nutrition Labeling and Education Act requires foods under FDA jurisdiction to bear nutrition labeling and requires food labels that bear nutrient content claims and health claims to comply with specific requirements.

Of the three concepts the FDA uses to describe its responsibility to the food system, "safe, wholesome and appropriately labeled," "wholesome" seems to be the most ill-defined by the FDA. Is a hydrogenated oil wholesome? Milk with rBST? Fat made out of synthetic chemicals? The FDA apparently thinks so, while we disagree. But fortunately, in most cases, good label reading will steer you clear of less desirable foods.

HOW TO READ AN INGREDIENTS LABEL

Ingredients are listed in the ingredients panel in descending order of predominance (weight). It matters, therefore, whether "sugar" is listed as the first or the last ingredient on the panel. If it is the first ingredient listed, then it is the primary ingredient in the product.

HOW TO READ A "NUTRITION FACTS" LABEL

Nutrition Facts labels are required on most food packages. Nutrition Facts will tell you the calories, fat, cholesterol, sodium, carbohydrate, protein, and some vitamins, in a designated serving size of a food product. It will also tell you the percent of Daily Value. Daily Value includes the recommended daily amounts (RDA) and the percentage of the ingredient found in the food. The percent of Daily Values found on a food label are based on a daily diet of two thousand calories. Your Daily Values may be higher or lower depending on your caloric needs.

Nutrition Facts

Serving Size 1 cup (228g)
Servings Per Container 2

Amount Per Serving

Calories 90   Calories from Fat 30

% Daily Value*

Total Fat 3g	**5%**
Saturated Fat 0g	**0%**
Cholesterol 5mg	**2%**
Sodium 280mg	**12%**
Total Carbohydrate 13g	**4%**
Dietary Fiber 6g	**24%**
Sugars 3g	
Protein 3g	

Vitamin A   80%   •   Vitamin C   60%

Calcium   4%   •   Iron   4%

* Percent Daily Values are based on a 2,000 calorie diet. Your daily values may be higher or lower depending on your calorie needs:

	Calories:	2,000	2,500
Total Fat	Less than	65g	80g
Sat Fat	Less than	20g	25g
Cholesterol	Less than	300mg	300mg
Sodium	Less than	2,400mg	2,400mg
Total Carbohydrate		300g	375g
Dietary Fiber		25g	30g

Calories per gram:

Fat 9   •   Carbohydrate 4   •   Protein 4

FDA RESTRICTIONS FOR TERMS SUCH AS "LOW-FAT" AND "LIGHT"

* "Fat free" means less than 0.5 gram of fat per serving.
* "Low fat" means 3 grams of fat or less per serving.
* "Light" (or "lite") means one-third of the calories or no more than one-half of the fat of the higher-fat version; or no more than one-half the sodium of the higher sodium version.
* "Cholesterol free" means less than 2 milligrams of cholesterol and 2 grams (or less) of saturated fat per serving.
* "Lightly salted" means 50 percent less sodium than is normally added to the food. (*Note*: The term *salt* is not synonymous with *sodium*, so phrases such as "no salt added" or "unsalted" are potentially misleading.
* "Sodium free" and "salt-free" mean less than 5 milligrams of salt per serving.
* "Low sodium" means 140 milligrams sodium or less per serving.
* "Calorie free" means less than five calories per serving.
* "Low calorie" means forty calories or less per serving.
* "High fiber" means 5 grams of fiber or more per serving.
* "Excellent" or "High source" of a nutrient is defined as supplying between 20 percent of the Daily Value of the nutrient.
* "Good source" of a nutrient is defined as supplying between 10 and 19 percent of the Daily Value of the nutrient.
* "Lean" meat, poultry, seafood, and packaged meats have less than 5 grams of fat, 2 grams of saturated fat, and 95 milligrams of cholesterol per serving size.

OTHER FDA REGULATIONS

* Fruit Juice: Under FDA labeling laws, if a product is "fruit juice sweetened" it must have characteristics of the fruit listed—i.e., a cereal listed as sweetened with apple juice must taste like apples. If the product is not characteristic of the fruit juice, then the product must be labeled as "modified or de-constituted fruit juice," meaning that the juice has

been stripped of its color and nutritional value leaving only sugar and water. "Stripped" juice cannot be labeled as juice.

❋ The claim "natural" means that "nothing artificial or synthetic (including all color additives regardless of source) has been included in, or has been added to, a food that would not normally be expected to be in the food."

❋ Foods are not allowed to be labeled as "fresh" if they have been treated with any form of preservatives. FDA guidelines state that when used in a manner which suggests that a food is unprocessed, the term *fresh* means that the food is in a raw state and has not been frozen or subjected to any form of thermal processing or preservation, except:

- Waxing raw fruits or vegetables with a wax approved by the FDA as a food additive
- Use of approved pesticides before or after harvest
- Pasteurization of milk
- Treatment of some raw foods with ionizing radiation.
- Treatment with milk chlorine wash or mild acid wash on produce
- Refrigeration

❋ "Fresh frozen" or "frozen fresh" means the food has been quickly frozen while still fresh. Appropriate blanching before freezing is permitted. "Quickly frozen" means freezing using a system such as blast-freezing (i.e., subzero Fahrenheit temperature with high-speed forced air directed at the food) for a sufficient length of time to freeze quickly to the center of the food with virtually no deterioration. Beware that it is not uncommon that some foods, such as poultry, partially thaw during transit and are sold as fresh. To avoid this, buy only frozen birds.

CLAIMS VERSUS LABELS

Believe labels, not claims on packaging, which can be deceptive. One example of a misleading claim on a package was found on a product labeled blueberry waffles. There were apparently no blueberries in the product at all. There are more subtly deceptive claims on packaging. Several so-called natural cereals, for instance, are loaded with refined sugar. The boxes may show bucolic country scenes, lavish color photographs of whole grains, fruits, nuts, pitchers of farm-fresh milk, and lazy cows. Forget all that and read the label, which tells the real story. Foods marketed and targeted for children are generally the least "whole." They often contain added sugar, artificial flavors, colors, and preservatives. Be wary of "kid-friendly" labels with bright colors and designs.

Do not assume that if you read a claim on a package, such as "natural flavors," all the contents are natural. In reality, only one ingredient may be "natural flavor." Or if you read the claim "fruit sweetened" on a box of cereal, for example, you might think you are escaping sugar. Not necessarily. Sugar might be an ingredient, too.

A–Z Guide to Finding Whole Foods Groceries

In the following guide, food products categories are listed alphabetically. Within most categories will be the following sections:

* *Best Choice* is the closest product found to be made of whole foods, with the fewest additives; but note that for some foods, there are no good choices and "None" is recommended.
* *Alert* lists additives or treatments of possible concern.
* *Other Concerns* or *General Concerns* is where commentary, when deemed appropriate, is presented about the product category.

Note: To avoid redundancy, we do not state "organic" for every "best choice," but we recommend certified organic whenever possible.

Also, please turn to chapter 2 for additives to avoid and more information on processed foods that may be itemized in an "alert."

BAKED GOODS AND BAKING SUPPLIES

General Guidelines: Look for whole grain breads and crackers such as whole wheat, corn, oats, barley, rice, amaranth, and rye. Make sure the words *whole wheat* are on food ingredients labels for wheat products. Look for whole grain baked goods with the fewest ingredients, such as whole wheat, water, leavening, salt.

Special Concerns: "Enriched flour" means that the flour has been stripped of much of its nutritional value, and vitamins have been added back in, in an attempt to compensate.

Alert: Many breads and crackers are made with refined flour, sugar, excessive salt, hydrogenated oils, artificial colors and flavors, dough conditioners, and preservatives.

Other Concerns: Read ingredients labels particularly carefully for baked goods such as boxed coffee cakes and doughnuts, as they can contain a great many additives. Baking mixes can contain hydrogenated oils, sugar, BHT, artificial color, artificial flavor, and preservatives. Breakfast toaster pastries can contain significant amounts of artificial colors and flavors. Highly seasoned products, such as croutons, may have a high fat content, and a number of artificial flavors. Read labels carefully!

Special Note about Flour: The best flour is that which has been milled at home (see chapter 6 for equipment recommendations), or freshly milled at a store. The reason for this is that the natural oils in freshly milled flour will not be rancid. If you buy packaged flour, buy small amounts at a time, and store in the freezer (see chapter 4). Make sure to buy whole grain flour—whole wheat, oat, brown rice, corn. "White" flour is not a whole grain flour. Unbleached white flour with germ means that the wheat germ has been removed from the grain, and then replaced. However, when wheat germ is exposed to air, its nutritional value diminishes considerably, and the oils in the germ can become rancid.

Note: Baking at home from scratch is the most healthful and environmentally preferable option.

Baking Powder

Best Choice: Baking powder without sodium aluminum sulfate.

General Concerns: Sodium aluminum sulfate. Although baking powder is not a major source of aluminum intake, and although aluminum has not been proven to cause Alzheimer's disease, high levels of aluminum have been found in the brains of people with Alzheimer's, so it's prudent to avoid aluminum whenever possible.

Note: Low-sodium baking powder uses potassium bicarbonate instead of sodium bicarbonate.

Sugar and Sweeteners

Best Choice: Maple syrup, honey, Sucanat, molasses, rice syrup, date sugar, barley malt, stevia, concentrated fruit juice.

Alert: Artificial colors.

General Concerns:

* The color of honey has to do with the flowers from which the bees harvested the nectar and isn't an indicator of nutritional content. However, the darker the color the more pungent the flavor.

* Avoid Canadian maple syrup, which may have been processed with formaldehyde-based tablets (outlawed in 1994, but still being used up by some) and any maple syrup that doesn't specifically say "Pure Maple Syrup." Or, buy certified organic maple syrup.

* Minute amounts of lead are found in some maple syrup. The cause is the lead solder found in older maple sugaring equipment. The syrup with the highest lead contamination seems to be from small hobby operations where the sap can sit in a tank for a day or two. Commercial operations move sap very fast, so their syrups are less likely to pick up lead.

* Some Sucanat has honey added for extra sweetness. Sucanat is sometimes labeled organic. (See chapter 4, "The Green Pantry," for more on Sucanat.)

Vanilla Extract

Best Choice: Real vanilla flavor (as opposed to artificially flavored).

Alert: Vanillin, an artificial flavor.

General Concerns: Always double-check the vanilla before you buy it in bulk; if it has a very pungent alcohol smell, it has turned bad. Please note, all liquid vanilla has alcohol in it, so even with fresh vanilla there is an alcohol smell, but with bad vanilla, the smell will be very, very strong. Pure vanilla extract may contain glycerin, propylene glycol, sugar dextrose, or corn syrup, and the content of ethyl alcohol is not less than 35 percent by volume. "Vanilla flavoring" means extract with *less* than 35 percent alcohol.

BEVERAGES

Coffee

Best Choice: Preferably organic coffee from shade-grown beans.

General Concerns: There are four ways to decaffeinate coffee. One way is "Swiss water processed," using pure water, and is the purest method available. Two methods of decaffeination use solvents— methylene chloride and ethyl acetate are the two solvents that have been approved for use in the United States by the FDA. Methylene chloride is a carcinogen. Ethyl acetate doesn't pose any risk to the consumer. The fourth method of decaffeination is water and carbon dioxide. If the label says "naturally decaffeinated" it will mean it was decaffeinated by either the Swiss water processed method, or the water and carbon dioxide method. The only way to find out which method was used is to call the company. Decaffeinated coffee manufactured in the United States is, for the most part, done through water processing.

> ✳ Avoid bleached filters, which may contain small amounts of dioxin. Buy unbleached coffee filters or a reusable gold filter instead.

Note: You can help protect migratory birds' winter home habitat by buying coffee made from shade-grown beans. Usually organic, the coffee comes from farms that use the traditional under-tree growing style, rather than the more recent, pesticide-intensive sun-grown method that destroys bird habitats. Shade-grown coffee provides habitats for migratory birds in Central and South America and Indonesia, as well as providing the fuller flavor of beans that have been slowly ripened.

Tea

Best Choice: Loose tea leaves, herbs.

General Concerns: When possible buy tea bags that have been made with unbleached cotton or paper. Artificial sweeteners.

Note: As with decaffeinated coffee, choose "naturally decaffeinated" tea.

Soda

Best Choice: Juice mixed with seltzer and only natural flavors.

Commonly Found Additives: Artificial color, artificial flavor, corn syrup, sugar, aspartame (NutraSweet or Equal), caffeine.

Other Concerns: The sugar content of sodas can be a staggering ten teaspoons per twelve-ounce can. Even some "natural" sodas contain fructose as a sweetener.

Instant Hot Chocolate or Cocoa

Best Choice: Whole cocoa bought in bulk or large tin.

Alert: Artificial flavors, artificial dyes, preservatives, hydrogenated oils.

Note: Most supermarkets do not carry whole food instant cocoa. Ask the manager to stock it, or find it instead at your health food store. Since cocoa is not naturally sweet, you may want to sweeten the cocoa at home with a whole food sweetener.

Syrups (Chocolate)

Best Choice: None.

Bottled Water

General Concerns: Bottled water, by FDA definition, is water that is sealed in bottles or other containers, and does not include mineral water or soda water. Bottled water must meet FDA regulations for trihalomethane, chloroform, and organic compounds. In addition it must meet standards of chemical quality and must not contain chemical substances and excess metals.

Juice

Fresh Juice

Best Choice: 100 percent fresh squeezed.

Alert: Watch out for added sugar. Look for a label that says "100 percent juice."

Frozen Concentrates

Best Choice: 100 percent pure juice.

Alert: A product label should read "no added sugar" if it is made from concentrate. Aspartame (NutraSweet, Equal).

Reconstituted Juice

Alert: If any water is added in excess of the amount of water needed to reconstitute the ingredient to single strength, the word *water* has to be listed in the ingredients statement.

Juice in Bottles, Aseptic Packages, Cans

Best Choice: 100 percent fruit juice.

Alert: Pay particular attention to see if the juice contains NutraSweet or Equal (aspartame).

General Alert: Watch out for juice "drinks," "cocktails," "fruit punches," and "fruit nectars." They can contain 10 percent juice or even less, and a full range of sweeteners and artificial flavors and colors.

CANNED GOODS

General Concerns: Avoid imported cans to ensure you do not expose yourself to lead soldering. While fine in a pinch, canned fruits and vegetables are not as nutritious as fresh or frozen. The interiors of some cans are lined in plastic and can leach hormone-disrupting materials into the food. See chapter 2 for more information. Read labels of canned soups carefully. Some brands can contain partially hydrogenated oils, sugar, sulfites, flavor enhancers, preservatives, and monosodium glutamate.

Baby Foods

Best Choice: Any plain jarred baby food, such as peaches, peas, carrots; plain boxed whole grain cereal. In choosing baby food it is particularly desirable to buy products that are certified organic.

Alert: Avoid combined jarred baby foods such as "chicken and pasta" or "apples and yogurt," since they are more likely to contain sugar, cornstarch, salt, rice starch. Avoid baby food "desserts," which are very likely to contain sugar.

Note: The best solution is to make your own, using organic fruits and vegetables.

Canned Processed Meats

Best Choice: Tuna fish, clams, chicken.
  Commonly Found Additives: Nitrates, salt.

Canned Tomatoes

Best Choice: Tomatoes, tomato juice, pulp (salt, citric acid).
  Alert: Hydrogenated oils.

  ❋ Most packers of tomato products effectively trim off, sort out, and discard rotten tomatoes. However, some mix rotten tomato products in with the healthy. The FDA defines these products as adulterated; however, since some slip through inspection, people with mold allergies should be particularly cautious about using canned tomato products.

CONDIMENTS, DRESSINGS, SPREADS

General Guidelines: When buying barbecue sauce, chili sauce, ketchup, and other condiments, read labels to avoid hydrogenated oils, preservatives, and artificial colors and flavors.

Mayonnaise

Best Choice: Substitute yogurt, or a low-fat alternative. Otherwise choose a mayonnaise with eggs, oil, and spices.
  Alert: Partially hydrogenated oils, preservatives.
  Other Concerns: High fat content.

Oils

Best Choice: Look for oils labeled "expeller pressed," "mechanically pressed," or in the case of olive oil, "cold-pressed." "Expeller-pressed" and "mechanically pressed" mean oil that has been extracted from the seed mechanically, as opposed to chemically. Another term for mechanically expressed oil is "unrefined."

Alert: Solvent extraction is a chemical method of extracting oil from seeds. Hexane is the most common chemical used in solvent extraction. Oils obtained through this process are considered to be refined oils. "Refined" oil may include anticlouding agents, BHT, BHA, and propyl gallate.

Other Concerns: "Cold-pressed" oil is misleading, since every oil (except olive oil, which can truly be cold-pressed) requires a temperature extraction level that seldom falls below 140°–160°F. The high temperature required, however, is not believed to result in a loss of nutrients or flavor. "Refined" oil is also often stripped of oil's naturally occurring vitamin E, which can act as a natural preventative against rancidity. The "best choice" oils contain this naturally occurring vitamin E.

* Unrefined oils can become rancid more quickly than refined oils, and should either be refrigerated or purchased in smaller quantities.

* When heated to too high a temperature, oils smoke and give off toxic fumes. (Please see chapter 4, "The Green Pantry," for specific oils and their smoke points.)

Of Interest: Sunflower and corn oil are the only oils indigenous to North America.

Olive Oil

Because olive oil comes from the soft pulp of the fruit rather than from a seed it needs no high pressure extraction and can truly be considered "cold-pressed."

Olives are crushed in a mill that breaks the pulp but not the pits. The first extraction is a gentle pressing that does not heat the oil much beyond room temperature. The oil is then separated from the olive water. Oil obtained from this first pressing is the only oil that can be called "virgin olive oil."

"Virgin" olive oil comes in three grades: "extra-virgin," "fine virgin," and "plain virgin." The differences are solely those of taste and acidity, with the "plain virgin" having the highest acid content and the "extra-virgin" having the lowest.

"Pure" olive oil is still 100 percent olive oil, but it is not "virgin." In other words, "pure olive oil" is extracted from second pressings, which require higher temperatures for extraction, reducing nutrient content, or solvent-extraction, which can leave a chemical residue.

Olives

Green

Best Choice: Olives, water, salt, sorbic acid.

Alert: Thickening agents, preservatives, salt.

Black

Best Choice: Olives, water, salt, or brine (ferrous glucanate, iron, used to retain color).

Alert: Preservatives, salt.

Jams and Jellies

Best Choice: Fruit (pectin, citric acid), no added sugar.

Note: See discussion of "fruit juice sweetened" on page 75. Aspartame (NutraSweet, Equal).

Pickles and Relishes

Best Choice: Cucumbers, peppers (salt or brine).

Alert: Salt, sulfiting agents, artificial colors.

Note: You have to look hard for pickles without artificial colors. If there are no acceptable brands in the traditional pickle aisle of your supermarket, try the dairy section or look elsewhere in the store for "kosher" dills, which are usually not dyed.

Salad Dressing

Best Choice: Oil, vinegar, spices, vegetables such as onion.

Alert: Fat, sulfites, salt, sugar, artificial flavors, and colors.

Vinegar (Distilled, Red/White Wine, Balsamic, Cider Vinegar)

Best Choice: 100 percent vinegar.

Alert: Sulfiting agents, for those who are allergic. Read the entire label scrupulously—some labels on balsamic vinegar, we discovered, listed sulfites in an obscure location.

DAIRY PRODUCTS

General Information

Organic Dairy Products: Organic milk is milk from cows that have been fed organic feed and have not been treated with synthetic pesticides, antibiotics, growth hormones, or other drugs. Certified organic milk and other dairy products are available in most parts of the country.

Pasteurization: Pasteurization heats milk to a high temperature to kill bacteria. This high heat does affect the composition of milk, allegedly destroying some nutrients. However, nearly all milk sold in America has been pasteurized.

Homogenization: Homogenization reduces the size of fat globules so that the milk doesn't have lumps.

rBST: Recombinant bovine growth hormone (rBGH or rBST) is a controversial bioengineered drug that is given to cows to increase milk production. See chapter 2, step 1, for more information. Most stores in the country carry at least one brand of milk from cows that have not been treated with rBST. Ask the manager to point out to you the specific brand, if you are unsure. Organic milk never comes from rBST-treated cows.

Organic Dairy Products: Certified organic milk and dairy products are currently available in most parts of the country.

Food Coloring: When a coloring has been added to butter, cheese, or ice cream, it does not need to be declared in the ingredients list unless it is a color additive that has special safety restrictions. Blue cheese often has blue and green dyes in it, for example, and blue and green dyes are often used to mask any yellowing in the curd of other dairy products. The FDA recommends voluntary declaration of all coloring. Dairy ingredients are often bleached with benzoyl peroxide or a mixture of benzoyl peroxide with potassium alum, calcium sulfate, and magnesium carbonate.

PCB Concentrations: The FDA allows residues of PCBs in dairy products to be 1.5 parts per million.

Vitamin Fortification: Farms often add the ingredients of vitamins A and D, although they are not required to by the FDA. Vitamin D is added for public health reasons, and vitamin A to replace that which could be lost due to exposure to light.

Low-Fat

Some foods labeled "light," "low-fat," or "nonfat" can be less whole—containing more stabilizers, preservatives, and artificial flavors—than their traditional counterparts. This is particularly true for foods labeled "nonfat." Cottage cheese and yogurt products are an example of a food where the "low-fat" version can be as whole as the full fat, but the nonfat version has preservatives and flavorings. Look for low-fat dairy products that do not contain chemical additives.

Butter

Best Choice: Organic cream and salt (optional).

Second choice: Nonorganic cream, salt (optional).

Alert: Saturated fat. Use sparingly. Butter can have added ingredients that are not on the label, such as preservatives, flavor, sweeteners, and dyes.

Note: To ensure the purest butter, buy from a dairy that doesn't use rBST and additives.

Cheese

Best Choice: Low-fat cheese, containing milk, cream, salt, rennet, cheese cultures.

Alert: Corn syrup, preservatives, sugar, food starch, artificial colors. Processed "cheese foods," processed cheeses, and "American" cheeses are likely to contain corn syrup, preservatives, and hydrogenated oils.

  ✳ Some cottage cheeses also contain sugar and food starches.

Other Concerns: As a rule of thumb, harder cheeses have less fat than softer cheeses.

Tip: Consider trying Quark cheese (German term for curds). It is a soft white cheese with a slightly acidic taste and smooth, spreadable texture. It is low in fat, sodium, and calories and derives only 30 percent of calories per serving from fat. Use it as a substitute for sour cream, cream cheese, Neufchâtel cheese, ricotta, and cottage cheese. Choose freshly made Quark, since its shelf life is about fourteen days from manufacture.

Chocolate Milk

Best Choice: Low-fat milk, cocoa, whole food sweetener such as Sucanat.

Alert: Sugar, corn syrup, artificial flavors and colors, preservatives.

Condensed or Evaporated Milk

Best Choice: None.

Alert: The processing causes a significant reduction of nutritional value.

Sweetened Condensed Milk

Best Choice: None.

Alert: Sugar, corn syrup, preservatives. The processing causes a significant reduction of nutritional value.

Cottage Cheese

Best Choice: Low-fat; dairy, whey salt, lecithin, enzymes.

Other Concerns: Cottage cheese with premixed fruit can have sugar, high-fructose corn syrup, aspartame (NutraSweet, Equal).

Cream Cheese

Best Choice: Low-fat cream cheese culture, salt.

Alert: Cream cheese labeled "light," "fat-free," or "soft" tends to have more additives, preservatives, and artificial flavors. Look carefully for the purest brand.

Dried Milk

Best Choice: Organic dried/powdered milk.

Alert: Added vitamins, emulsifiers, preservatives. Processing significantly reduces nutritional value.

Ice Cream and Frozen Yogurt

Best Choice: Low-fat ice cream and yogurts; fruit sorbet as a more healthful substitute.

Other Concerns: Among traditional ice cream and frozen yogurt brands there is a wide range, from great whole food choices, containing just the essential ingredients—cream and sugar—to those containing many additives, a lot of sugar, and preservatives. Aspartame (NutraSweet, Equal).

Instant Coffee Creamers, Nondairy Creamers

Best Choice: None.

Alert: Corn syrup solids, partially hydrogenated oils, artificial flavor, preservatives. Contains casinine, a milk product; fats.

Margarine

Best Choice: None.

Alert: Hydrogenated or partially hydrogenated oils.

Milk

Best Choice: 100 percent pasteurized low-fat cow's or goat's milk.

Commonly Found Additives: Vitamin D_3 (a necessary nutrient added to milk for public health reasons).

Other Concerns:
* Allergies: Milk is a very common allergen.
* Milk has a high fat content. Choose low-fat when possible.
* Choose rBST-free milk when possible.

Sour Cream

Best Choice: Cultured cream, whey, enzymes.

Alert: Make sure that you don't choose a sour cream substitute by mistake.

Other Concerns: See Cream Cheese.

Yogurt

Best Choice: Yogurt containing milk (preferably skim), yogurt cultures, whole fruit, fruit juice sweetener.

Alert: Yogurts range widely from those containing just milk, yogurt cultures, and plain fruit or fruit juices to yogurts containing many additives and sugar. Notice that some yogurts contain aspartame (NutraSweet or Equal).

Eggs

Best Choice: Eggs from free-range hens that have not been treated with antibiotics and have been raised on organic feed.

Alert: All eggs should be cooked thoroughly, as the deadly bacterium *Salmonella enteritidis* is found in raw eggs, including high-grade eggs.

* The FDA's acceptable limit of PCBs in eggs is 0.3 part per million.
* Eggs do not have to be dated if they have not been graded by the USDA. Eggs do not have to be graded unless they come from a farm of more than three thousand hens or the producer sells eggs from more than one farm. The USDA recommends eating eggs within three weeks of purchase. As long as the eggs remain refrigerated, within the three weeks the eggs only diminish in quality rather than becoming unsafe to eat.

Note: Look for eggs from free-range hens; they have most likely not been raised in a confined factory farm.

DRIED GOODS

General Guidelines: Read labels for the additives of concern outlined in chapter 2. You will find some of these additives in unexpected places. Chili spice powder can contain sulfites, for example. Applesauce can contain artificial colors and even hydrogenated oils.

Cereal

Best Choice: Whole grains such as wheat, corn, or oats, without sweetener, or sweetened with whole foods sweetener.

Note: "Puffed" cereal is the least nutritious because high temperatures are used to "puff" the grain kernel, destroying some vitamins and minerals in the process.

Alert: Because most granolas have a lot of oil in them, you should refrigerate or freeze your granola to keep it from going rancid, if you are buying a large quantity that won't be used in a week or so. Make sure to store the granola in an airtight container or a well-sealed plastic bag to keep it fresh.

General Concerns: Sugar, corn syrup, artificial colors, partially hydrogenated oils, aspartame (NutraSweet or Equal), artificial flavors, preservatives, BHT added to cereal.

Herbs

General Concern: Ask your health food stores how quick the turnover is for the dried herbs sold in bulk. Quick turnovers offer you a better chance of buying a fresh product. Smell the herbs to check for staleness. Air and light destroy an herb's or spice's freshness, therefore it is best to buy the herb in its whole-leaf state, since crumbling the herb releases the essential oils that give the herb its flavor. The same goes for spices; buy those that aren't preground.

Alert: Ask your store manager to label any herbs that have been irradiated.

Nuts

General Concerns: When the oils in nuts go rancid the nuts should not be eaten. Make sure nuts are fresh and avoid any that are discolored, shriveled, rubbery, obviously moldy, or taste stale. If you buy nuts in bulk, ask the store for permission to taste a sample before buying in quantity.

* Aflatoxin: Be particularly vigilant about avoiding stale or rancid peanuts and peanut butter because the carcinogenic mold aflatoxin can grow on moldy nuts. Other nuts vulnerable to aflatoxin are almonds, Brazil nuts, pecans, pistachios, and walnuts. If you grind nut butter in the store, make sure the machine is thoroughly cleaned before you proceed.

* Buy only whole nuts, rather than sliced, or chopped. Whole nuts store well, but when they are sliced or broken, their oily flesh is exposed to air and can become rancid quicker. Avoid "slivered" almonds, as they are particularly vulnerable to rancidity.

"Plain" Nuts

Best Choice: 100 percent nuts.

Alert: Corn oil (the container is coated in oil), artificial coloring (in the case of red pistachios), salt.

Roasted Nuts

Best Choice: 100 percent nuts.

Alert: Hydrogenated oils, flavor enhancers, salt, thickening agents.

Dry Roasted Nuts

Best Choice: 100 percent nuts (spices).

Alert: Salt, corn syrup, flavor enhancers.

Note: Other than plain nuts, these are the most healthful, without added oil and salt.

Nut Butters

Best Choice: Freshly ground nuts, such as peanuts.

Alert: Partially hydrogenated oils, corn syrup, sugar, dextrose, stabilizers, salt.

Note: For freshness, your best choice is to buy nut butters in a store that will grind them on the spot. However, make sure that the machine is cleaned daily, to avoid the mold aflatoxin.

Pasta

Best Choice: 100 percent unrefined durum semolina; brown rice, kamut, corn.

Concerns: You have to look hard to find whole grain pasta. Most has been refined and enriched.

Prepared Coatings

Bread Crumbs

Best Choice: Whole grain flours, leavening, salt, spices.

Alert: Dough conditioners, flavor enhancers, preservatives, partially hydrogenated oils.

Other Concerns: High fat content.

Shake-in-a-Bag Types

Best Choice: Herbs and spices.

Alert: Hydrogenated oils, flavor enhancers, preservatives.

Meat Glazes

Best Choice: None.

Alert: Flavor enhancers, thickening agents, sugar, corn syrup.

Instant Potatoes

Best Choice: None.

Rice (Brown, Enriched, Converted, White)

Best Choice: Whole, brown rice—long, medium, or short grain.

Commonly Found Additives: Read the labels of seasoned rice carefully to see if the products contain flavor enhancers, preservatives, and stabilizers.

Other Concerns:

* White rice: When rice is polished and milled to create white rice, many nutrients are lost.
* Instant rice is the least nutritious.
* Enriched rice returns some, but not all, of the nutrients.
* Converted rice, sometimes called parboiled, is the most nutritious option of the processed rices and is steamed and pressurized before milling, forcing 70 percent of the nutrients of the bran and germ into the grain, although the fiber remains unaffected.

Stuffing Mix

Best Choice: Whole grain flour, natural leavening, spices, butter.

Alert: High salt and fat content. Flavor enhancers, dough conditioners, preservatives, partially hydrogenated oils.

Salt

Best Choice: Sea salt made from evaporated seawater, with added iodine (and dextrose to stabilize the iodine).

General Concerns: Although purists would not agree with us that iodized sea salt is the best choice, we choose this because iodine helps prevent thyroid diseases. Since iodine is often undersupplied in the diet, if it is added to the salt you buy, it is an insurance your family may be getting enough. However, some think that because iodine is now so prevalent in salt we may be getting too much iodine. Kosher salt is another good alternative. It does not contain any additives, including iodine.

Note: To reduce your overall salt intake and help prevent hypertension, substitute for salt spicy flavorings such as garlic, ginger, or herb blends.

FRESH PRODUCE

Waxes and Coatings: Everyone is familiar with the apple or pepper that has a glossy, oily shine, indicating that the fruit or vegetable has been waxed. Numerous fruits, vegetables, and nuts receive a wax coating that may not be so identifiable, such as that found on eggplants, grapefruit, grapes, or tomatoes. When these waxes are mixed with pesticides, the pesticides cannot be washed off. (Many pesticides are systemic and can't be washed off anyway.) It is federal law that retailers prominently display a sign identifying fresh fruits and vegetables that are treated with postharvest wax or resin coating. The sign must read "coated with food-grade animal-based wax, to maintain freshness," or the phrase "coated with food-grade vegetable-, petroleum-, beeswax-, and/or shellac-based wax or resin, to maintain freshness" as appropriate. Make sure the stores you shop at display such a sign. Only buy waxed produce that can be peeled.

Adulterated Produce: It has been the practice of some growers, packers, and distributors of yellow varieties of sweet potatoes to artificially color the skins of such potatoes with a red dye. The FDA now deems these sweet potatoes "adulterated." Report any such sweet potatoes to the produce manager. (If you cut them open and find the inside to be yellow, and the outside red, the sweet potatoes are suspect.)

Irradiated Produce: Food irradiation to kill bacteria has been approved in the United States on various foods, including fruit and vegetables. Ask your produce manager to label irradiated produce.

Bioengineered Produce: Genetic engineering permits scientists to develop plants that would never occur naturally. A flounder and a tomato can't naturally breed, of course, but scientists can use genetic engineering techniques to insert genes from a flounder into a tomato.

As of the end of 1994, the U.S. Department of Agriculture had approved more than 1,100 field trials of genetically engineered crops. Close to market are potatoes, tomatoes, corn, soybeans, squash, and cotton (some grown for cottonseed oil). A major health concern about genetic engineering is that the new products may cause susceptible individuals to become allergic to foods they previously could safely consume. The FDA's policy on bioengineering only requires labeling of these foods under certain exceptional circumstances. And the decision whether safety questions exist is left to the food manufacturers.

Buying Tips

Organic Produce: Look on the label or the package for evidence that the product is certified organic by a third party, either a government or a private certifier. This is the only guarantee that it is organic. There will likely be a difference in appearance between organic and conventional produce. Organic produce may vary in size, be less perfect in shape or coloring, or may be mottled. Note that chemicals used for nonorganic produce are used not just to eliminate bugs, but also for cosmetic purposes—such as to prevent a blemish on the skin of the fruit or vegetable. A Cornell researcher estimates that from 10 to 20 percent of insecticides and fungicides are applied simply to comply with strict cosmetic standards.

Organic produce may be more perishable than conventional produce. The fact that it may not be waxed makes it more easily dehydrated. It's also generally picked closer to ripeness, therefore reducing its shelf life. Lettuce, tomatoes, and beans should be eaten within a few days of purchase. Slightly wilted produce can be perked up by soaking it in cold water. Organic or conventional, one should be able to keep storable foods—potatoes, apples, beets, oranges, grapefruits, sweet potatoes—for a month or more in the refrigerator without any problem. Be careful to check for molds; they can form on fruits during long-term storage.

Produce Grown in the United States: Possibly the most important question we should be asking our produce manager is, "Where are these apples from?" or "Where did you get those berries?" Produce from very humid climates may be grown with heavier use of fungicides. Other countries often don't have the same level of pesticide controls as the United States—and in some cases we may even be importing produce that's been treated with chemicals banned in the United States. This circulating across borders of banned pesticides—including the practice by U.S. companies of selling U.S.-banned pesticides to Third World countries—has been called the "circle of poison." Retailers aren't required to label produce by its country of origin, but it would be useful for consumers if they did. It also would be easy for retailers to disclose this information, since shippers are required to declare it on shipping containers.

Locally Grown: Because they haven't been shipped long distances, local foods are less likely to have been treated with postharvest fungicides.

Exotic Produce: Exotic fruit, for example from the South Pacific, will add a sort of variety to one's diet, but that it had to travel eight thousand miles to get here should give one pause. And more than likely, that particular variety of fruit, which was the most commercially acceptable and able to withstand long-distance travel, has probably been favored in that marketplace at the expense of other local varieties that may be tastier or more nutritious.

* *First Best Choice:* Locally grown, organic, in season, unpackaged; variety and diversity. Hydroponics (vegetables grown in water; read label of produce carefully to determine if it is also organic).

* *Second Best Choice:* Grown in the United States, no waxes and chemicals such as postharvest fungicides.

* *Alert:* No information available as to where it is grown; waxed; sprayed with fungicides; imported; exotic; imported or shipped many thousands of miles; out-of-season produce; bioengineered or irradiated produce. The farther away the food was grown, the more likelihood of high concentrations of postharvest chemicals.

Salad Bar

Best Choice: Raw or steamed fresh fruit and vegetables.

Alert: Dressings, prepared salads, and pastas full of fat and additives.

Note: Unless the ingredients of the available salad dressings are labeled and you can determine the extent of the additives and fat, either buy your own bottle of additive-free dressing, or make it from vinegar and oil.

(Sulfiting agents are no longer used on most salad bars.)

FROZEN FOODS

General Guidelines: The simpler the food, the less processed it will be. For example, buy plain vegetables as opposed to vegetable mixes. If the food package claims "organic" then the chance of unwanted additives is lower.

Alert: BHT is added to some frozen foods. Read labels carefully to see if nitrates are included in the ingredients list (and if they are, pass up the product). Products such as french fries can contain monosodium glutamate (MSG) and preservatives.

* Some frozen vegetables such as peas and lima beans can have substantial amounts of salt because the vegetables have been processed in a salt brine before freezing. If this process has been used, the salt must be listed on the label.

Special Concerns: Try to determine where the frozen foods are packaged. A local packer, for example, might utilize locally produced fruits and vegetables, thereby reducing transport costs.

MEAT AND FISH

Best Choice: Free-range meats or poultry products raised without antibiotics or growth stimulants, fed organic feed, and raised on a sustainable farm. Look for "raising claim" labels that explicitly state that the meat is raised with certified organic feed and/or without antibiotics or other feed additives, and that the grazing area has not been sprayed.

* "Natural" means meat or poultry products are minimally processed and contain no artificial additives such as preservatives, artificial colors or flavors. The "minimally processed" claim is an empty one, though, because meat is not a processed food.
* "Free-range" does not necessarily mean drug-free.
* "Organic": Currently, the USDA prohibits meat and poultry from being labeled as organically produced. However, there are organic livestock standards, and some farms follow these.

Other Concerns: Bacterial contamination of meat by salmonella and other bacteria is a serious health problem. Make sure to use soap and hot water to clean all of the surfaces that have come into contact with the meat.

Cold Cuts (Bologna, Chicken, Corned Beef, Ham, Liverwurst, Pastrami, Pepperoni, Roast Beef, Salami, Turkey)
Best Choice: Nitrate-free whole turkey or chicken breast cooked and sliced.

Alert: BHT, BHA, other preservatives, nitrites, excessive salt, fat.

Fish and Shellfish

Safest Choice: Farm-raised fish is a safer choice, since the farm environment is isolated from pollution sources. For fresh "wild" fish, contact your local Department of Fisheries, which can provide you with "eating advisories."

Other Concerns: Pollution contamination. The marine environment suffers from pollution and habitat destruction, leading to the loss of several million tons of edible marine fish a year. Fish can accumulate fat-soluble pesticides like DDT; industrial chemicals like PCBs and dioxins; and toxic metals like mercury. Clams and oysters can accumulate lead and cadmium. Chemical contamination of fish is a serious problem; those most at risk are pregnant women and children.

Never buy imported shellfish. The risk of bacterial contamination is too great, due to poor handling and irregular refrigeration practices. Ask your grocer to specifically label where shellfish and fish come from.

> ✽ The FDA allows PCBs in fish at concentrations of two parts per million.

Canned Tuna Fish

Best Choice: Tuna packed in water, no added salt or oil.

Other Concerns: Look for the labels saying "dolphin safe" to be sure that dolphins haven't been caught in the tuna nets.

Hot Dogs

Best Choice: "Uncured turkey frankfurter." Or skip meat altogether by choosing soy/tofu dogs with spices.

Alert: Even chicken frankfurters labeled "healthy" and "low-fat" may contain corn syrup and nitrites.

SNACKS

General Guidelines: Snacks are notoriously high in fat and sugar. Try to reduce consumption of "junk food" as much as possible by substituting whole food snacks such as fresh fruit.

Candy

Best Choice (Best Compromise): Maple sugar candy. Candy made with natural dyes instead of synthetic.*

Alert: Artificial colors, hydrogenated oils, aspartame (NutraSweet or Equal).

Dried Fruit

Best Choice: 100 percent dried fruit.

Alert: Sulfiting agents.

* Some fruit may have added sugar.
* Banana chips may be fried.

Note: Nonsulfered fruit will be less plump and darker in color; however, it will still be very flavorful.

Chips

Best Choice: Potatoes, corn, or grains (lime, oil, salt).

Alert: The more flavored the chip, the more likely it contains a high number of chemical additives.

* Partially or hydrogenated oils, artificial flavor, food dyes, monosodium glutamate (MSG).

Other Concerns: Choose reduced fat (baked, not fried, is best) and salt-free chips.

"Fruit Snacks"

Best Choice: Fruit, water, lemon juice.

Alert: Artificial colors and flavors, sulfites, mineral oil.

Other Concerns: Often packaged with the phrase "Snacks Made with Fruit," these products are sold in the breakfast section next to breakfast bars and cereals. Many "fruit snacks" have negligible fruit and large quantities of artificial colors and flavors.

---

*Health food stores and green supermarkets have increasing varieties of colored candies that have been dyed with vegetable and fruit juices, which are preferable to synthetic dyes.

Puddings, Gelatin Desserts

Best Choice: Real flavor and color; puddings made with whole grains.

    Alert: Artificial flavors and colors, preservatives.

Trail Mix

Best Choice: Nuts, seeds, unsulfured dried fruit.

    Alert: Sulfiting agents.

SOY PRODUCTS

Soy Cheese

Alert: Soy cheeses can contain casein, a milk derivative. (This can be of concern to someone who is eating soy cheese in an effort to avoid dairy products due to allergy.)

Soy Milk

Alert: Some soy milks have high fat content, but because they are made from soybeans, most of the fat is unsaturated. Most soy milk companies are producing lower fat varieties of their soy milk, and a few are unsweetened.

    Manufacturers are now fortifying soy milks with calcium and vitamin D in order to make a nutritionally comparable alternative to fortified milk.

Tofu

Best Choice: Tofu, well water (spices). You can choose tofu textured "firm," "silken," or "soft."

    Alert: Tofu is highly perishable, and it is very important that the tofu you buy is fresh (unhealthful microorganisms grow on souring tofu). Tofu that is "off" has a sour taste and should be discarded. It also feels slimy. Wash tofu every day and cover with fresh spring-water. Studies have shown that tofu that is sold in sealed packages has the lowest bacteria count.

Only buy tofu in bulk if it meets these conditions:

* It is covered with filtered water or springwater.
* It is kept in a cooler and is handled by store employees only. If the tofu is kept in a deli section, with cheeses, etc., make sure it is not in the deli case, since most deli cases are kept at 50°F and tofu should be kept at no higher than 41°F.
* If the tofu is kept in a self-serve bucket, make sure the store changes the water every day.
* If the water is discolored or yellow, do not buy the tofu.

MISCELLANEOUS

"Diet" Foods

Best Choice: None.

Alert: Partially hydrogenated oils, artificial flavors, artificial colors, aspartame, saccharin, emulsifiers, stabilizers.

ALTERNATIVE WAYS OF FINDING WHOLE FOODS

It can be exciting to step aside from shopping exclusively in conventional food stores and find food in other ways. In fact, you may find the most economical and abundant sources of whole, organic foods year-round are found outside of supermarkets. And there are unexpected rewards in alternative shopping, not the least of which is reconnecting with the natural world, the seasons, and learning how your food is grown.

When food is grown on your land, or by farmers you know, spring becomes equated with tender shoots of asparagus, strawberries, and rhubarb; and the dog days of August are passed by eating freshly picked, succulent cucumbers. The bounty of early fall is marked by an abundance of tomatoes and zucchini, and winter is heralded in with hearty soups made from harvested root vegetables. All of this connects you to your community and gives you a sense of your place on earth.

From a strictly practical point of view, finding food in farmers' markets, food co-ops, and other ways listed below can save you an enormous amount of money. Many people have found that though buying fresh organic food in supermarkets and health food stores can be prohibitively expensive, obtaining produce through alternative methods can be cheaper.

Alternative ways for acquiring food—such as CSAs and farmers' markets—bring us into close contact with the farmers as well as the seasons. Providing food that has often been picked freshly that morning, and sold from the back of their trucks, growers can chat with us about how the weather is affecting the crops and how the growing season is going, which helps to root us in our natural world. Finding food in alternative places is more social than shopping in a supermarket. You may meet new people, establish a social network, and feel a valuable sense of community.

A little creativity in finding organic food can reap rewards. I live in a rural community and buy organic produce eight months a year from a retired couple who are ardent organic gardeners. My family's enjoyment of the in-season fruits and vegetables that we get each week has renewed our interest in cooking because the food is so delicious. My daughter sees how her food is produced, even smells the soil where it is grown, and sees the cows that provide the milk. This enriches all of our lives.

FARMERS' MARKETS/GREEN MARKETS

There are no simple answers to preserving farms and agriculture, but so far, Farmers' Markets have been the most incredible solution going.

—Elizabeth Ryan, co-owner of Breezy Hill Orchards

Farmers' markets (also known as green markets) are returning to towns and cities everywhere. In fact, according to the USDA, 17,555 farmers' markets opened in the last decade, whereas twenty years ago there were only 100. Farmers' markets are treasured by farmers and consumers alike. Found deep in the middle of the largest cities, and in smaller towns across America, farmers' markets are usually outdoors and always colorful and festive. There local farmers, bakers, and food-based cottage industries set up in a communal area, once or twice a week or more, to sell their food to their community.

Most farmers' markets sell not only local organic produce but also local freshly baked goods such as scones, baguettes, focaccia; clotted cream and organic milk in glass bottles from local dairy farms; fiery salsas made from local tomatoes; ranch-raised ducks, chickens, and turkeys; and, of course, produce—basil, cilantro, mesclun, tomatoes, greens, scallions, lettuce of every sort, peppers, apples, pears, and melons. The variety is dependent only on the season. Farmers' markets provide the opportunity for farmers and consumers to meet in person, and it isn't uncommon for friendships between the two to develop over the course of a season's harvest. These old-fashioned gathering places are popping up across the country, but if you don't have one in your community, call your county's agriculture extension agent, or your state agriculture department, to inquire about the feasibility of establishing one.

To find a farmers' market near you, contact the following organizations. If there isn't a farmers' market in your area, join with friends and start one! Contact local farmers' organizations to determine whether there is enough interest.

* The USDA puts out an annual directory of farmers' markets.
* Farm Verified Organic Inc., RR 1, Box 40A, Medina, ND 58467.
* California Certified Organic Farmers, 303 Potrero Street, Suite 51, Santa Cruz, CA 95060.
* Organic Trade Association, P.O. Box 1078, 20 Federal Street #3, Greenfield, MA 01302.

CSAs

WHAT IS A CSA?

Joining a CSA is the next best thing to having your own garden. "CSA" means community-supported agriculture, which means a community of people supporting a local garden or farm either by work or by paying a share of expenses, and thereby becoming entitled to a season's fresh fruits and vegetables (or more, such as milk and honey, depending on the CSA). The CSA can either have an arrangement with a particular farm, or they can lease farmland and hire their own gardener or farmer to work it.

There are probably as many formulas for how to run a CSA as there are CSAs (there are hundreds around the country). Some CSAs are very strict proponents of biodynamic farming—that which follows the basic principles of nature and as defined by Rudolf Steiner (see Bio-dynamic Farming and Gardening Association in "Resources."). These CSAs are farm-centered, meaning that they are part of an established farming philosophy, one that is often biodynamic but usually at least organic and sustainable. By being members of such a farm's CSA, you help ensure the farm's economic viability. In one case we know of a farmer who needed a guaranteed local outlet for his produce in order to keep the farm afloat, and by developing a CSA, the farm survived.

Other CSAs are simply loosely woven groups of people who share an organic garden, its work and expenses. The group pools resources to lease or rent land, hires a farmer or gardener (or shares in the gardening), handles administrative jobs, and as a result the members are entitled to their share's worth of a season's harvest, usually twenty weeks of fruits and vegetables.

The great benefit of being a member of a CSA is a season's supply of freshly picked fruits and vegetables that are both economical and usually organic. It also can be a way for people in a community to support family farms in the vicinity. Because most CSAs require the person's share of expenses to be paid up front so the farmer/gardener can buy seeds and other equipment, there is some risk of losing the investment if there is a bad drought or flood. But realistically, the risk of losing the entire investment is slight.

BASIC RESPONSIBILITIES OF CSAs

The first job in starting a CSA is to form a membership core. From that core group other members are added by advertising and by word of mouth. Once the group has been established, the next step is to determine the group's vision. Decisions need to be made about the kind of farming the group wants to support, be it biodynamic, organic, or conventional. The parameters need to be established too. Is the CSA going to grow just vegetables? Fruits and berries? Are animals going to be involved for milk and meat, hens for eggs, bees for honey?

Shares in CSAs vary from group to group and sometimes have a sliding scale for low-income families. The cost of a share is usually determined by the CSA's budget, which includes the cost of seeds, salary for the farmer or gardener, and administrative expenses. The price of a share often works out to be comparable to the cost of nonorganic produce at the supermarket.

Arranging a CSA often means forging a partnership with a farm. In these instances, the farm often sets up the CSA, and the consumer finds out about it through the grapevine or from an advertisement. The group does not need to search for farmland. For CSAs that develop independently of a farm, finding appropriate land with healthy soil is a critical issue. Whereas leasing agricultural land can be cheap, it is important to lease land with a long-term lease, so all the work of developing and maintaining healthy soil is rewarded. A helpful clearinghouse of information for farmers, gardeners, and apprentices is Community-Supported Agriculture of North America (CSANA; see "Resources").

Besides actual farming, other jobs that need to be attended to by CSA members include administrative work such as bookkeeping, membership update mailings, and writing newsletters. If you want to find a CSA near you, a first step is to call your local Department of Agriculture, or your cooperative extensions, to see if there are any. Another avenue is to call Robyn Van En, author of *Basic Formula to Create Community Supported Agriculture,* or the Biodynamic Farming and Gardening Association, which has a database of five hundred CSAs in North America. They will send a free brochure, "Farm Supported Communities." See "Resources."

SUBSCRIPTION FARMING

If you know of a local farm whose produce and/or other products you would like to buy throughout the harvest season, but don't want as formal a relationship as a CSA, you may want to establish a "subscription" membership to the farm. Usually established on a weekly prepaid basis, with a subscription you commit to buying a set amount of food from one farm and thereby ensure a constant supply. This system is similar to a CSA, but there isn't any risk (you only pay as you go) or organizational obligations. Of course there isn't the degree of savings as you would have with a CSA, or the same entitlement to the food. For example, the farm may have melt-in-your-mouth strawberries, but they may use them all up themselves to make jam. Finding farms that have a subscription system isn't an easy task. If you find one, treasure it!

As with CSAs and cooperatives, there is nothing rigid about how subscription farms are established. Some get their produce every harvest season by adding their name to the list of consumers a local farm will sell to. As soon as it is available they buy food throughout the season, paying as they go. The arrangement is no more formal than that.

FOOD CO-OPS AND COOPERATIVE-BUYING CLUBS

The National Cooperative Business Association (NCBA) describes food-buying clubs and co-ops as "typically informal groups organized to buy directly from a wholesaler and save substantially on groceries."

Group members order in bulk and divide their order among themselves. Each person also volunteers time towards the tasks of ordering, bookkeeping, and distribution. Cooperative buying clubs may be organized to obtain common grocery items or special types of products such as produce, natural foods, or canned goods.

In some states the word *co-op* can apply only to those organizations that are legally incorporated. In those states, many "co-ops" are technically not co-ops but food-buying clubs that are cooperatively organized.

Food co-ops and buying clubs usually need to buy around four hundred dollars' worth of groceries a month to have access to the discounted prices of a co-op wholesaler. Just two or three households could meet that requirement easily. Most buying clubs work on a preorder and pay-on-delivery system, although some prepay when the order is submitted to the wholesaler.

You can save a lot of money on your food budget by buying food through a wholesale distributor, especially the more boxed cases of food the group is able to buy and split. You also save by not going to the grocery store as much—gas money or time, depending on where you live.

Two cooperative buying clubs have been big parts of my life, and they are as different as the sun and the moon, thereby good examples of the spectrum of possibilities of the cooperative system. One, the Hanover Food Co-operative, began in the early 1940s in a small New England town. Initiated by a group of young Dartmouth College professors and their families, it started off in a garage. It has long since grown to become a large food store, beloved by the entire community, and a much valued gathering place. Still a cooperative, the organization not only operates a large cooperative grocery store, but also a credit union and even an automotive service station. The cooperative bought land, some of which is used for a farmers' market, and other plots for individual gardens. When shopping, members provide the checkout clerk with a computerized card with their membership number, which is used to track the members' expenditures during the year. Every spring each member receives a check whose amount is determined by the cooperative's profits as well as by a percentage of the member's purchases for the year. The Hanover Food Co-operative is a socially responsible business with excellent employee benefits, and it is committed to marketing food grown and produced in the surrounding community. It also is an educational hub, offering cookbooks and services for the community such as bulletins about the environment, healthful food, and recycling. Would that we could all establish one of these in our communities!

The other food cooperative in my life, Green Squash (named by a five-year-old), is very low-key by comparison. A preorder food-buying cooperative, it consists of ten families who have very little extra time but manage to spare one night a month to get together for a potluck dinner, and find other time to collate orders, do book-keeping, and divide up deliveries. All of the members of the cooperative enjoy the sociability as well as saving money on monthly food bills.

HOW TO SET UP A SMALL FOOD CO-OP

How to Find Wholesalers and Other Resources

To find a local co-op wholesaler or existing buying clubs in your area, a helpful resource is Co-op Directory Services (see "Resources"). Also, the NCBA sells a video called *How to Start a Co-op Food Buying Club* that may be of help, as well as a book, *Starting Out Right: Guidelines for Organizing a New Retail Cooperative* (see "Resources").

Membership

With a small core membership, develop the co-op and establish a vision. Once you have determined the size you want the co-op to be, solicit members through word of mouth, advertising, and the like. Assign key positions: bookkeeper, order compiler, networker for delivery dates or potluck dinners, and those who meet the delivery truck.

General Procedures

Locate a wholesale distributor. Order monthly catalogs from the distributor, complete with sales fliers. Then . . .

1. Compile individual orders.
2. Compile communal bulk orders for cases. (Green Squash handles this every month at an "auction" time at their potluck suppers.)
3. Compile the entire group's order on one form and send to the wholesale distributor. (This is easiest if the system is computerized.)
4. Contact the distributor for delivery dates.

5. Meet the truck, and divide the order.
6. Refund money to members for back-ordered merchandise.
7. Make sure that everyone knows the dates for order dead-
   lines and potluck dinners. (In Green Squash this job rotates
   every month, and during a person's tenure he or she is
   called the "Sovereign.")

PICK-YOUR-OWN FARMS

In most states, the department of agriculture will provide you with
a brochure listing all pick-your-own farms in your state, county by
county. Some pick-your-own farms specialize in one particular fruit
or vegetable, such as apples or pumpkins. Trips to these kinds of
farms can become seasonal family traditions, to pick a bushel of
apples in the fall for instance. Other farms may provide an evolving
list of fruits and vegetables you can pick yourself throughout the
growing season, often beginning with strawberries in June and end-
ing with cut-your-own Christmas trees in December. Pick-your-
own farms are fun but don't necessarily save customers either time
or money.

MAIL-ORDER CATALOGS

A great deal of whole, organic food can be bought through the mail:
everything from dairy products like cheese; to fresh bread; to weekly
deliveries of organic produce baskets and organic meats. There are
hundreds of mail-order catalogs. Buying your family's groceries
through the mail can open up an entire array of healthful options for
those of you who have difficulty finding in your community a local
outlet for wholesome, freshly picked organic foods, or ranch-raised
meats. You can order weekly shipments to be delivered overnight.
Usually the produce is picked the morning it is shipped.

Packaged organic food is readily available through the mail too.
In fact, some co-op wholesalers will even ship orders with no min-
imum, via UPS, for those who don't want to start a buying club. See
"Resources" for some sources of catalogs.

GROWING YOUR OWN FOOD

Gardens are places to renew yourself in mind and body, to reawaken to the truth and beauty of the natural world, and to feel the life force inside and around you. And the organic way to garden is safer, cheaper, and more satisfying. Organic gardeners have shown that it's possible to have pleasant and productive gardens in every part of this country without using toxic chemicals. They make their home grounds an island of purity.

—Robert Rodale, founder of the Rodale Press, and
considered the father of organic gardening

There is nothing like the feeling of accomplishment that comes with picking a home-grown tomato a few yards away from the kitchen door, or picking the salad greens and herbs for the evening's meal. Watching the plants grow, from seed to fruition, is a source of wonder to the whole family. But most important, gardens are a great source of food.

Teaching you how to garden is beyond the scope of this book—nor would we presume to be experts. But there are a few guidelines we can offer, the most important of which is to get a really good book on the subject—*Rodale's Encyclopedia of Organic Gardening* is one. Talk to friends who garden, as they will be full of advice. Start small, making your first garden no bigger than you can comfortably handle. Select heirloom seeds (see chapter 2). Grow food that you like.

FORAGING

Native Americans had a diet of plants that most of us have never heard of. From agarita, alpine strawberry, American turk's cap lily, and arrow grass, to white oak, wild calla, woolly milk vetch, and yellow wild indigo, their food was a rich diversity of native plants.

But now their knowledge has become obscure. Fortunately, however, there are a number of expert foragers around the country, and we can learn a great deal from them.

Herbalist and nutritionist Deborah Lee is the most remarkable tour guide we can imagine to introduce us to the wonders of foraging. She overflows with inspiring wisdom about the natural world. Author of *Exploring Nature's Uncultivated Garden*, Lee has such a commonsense view of the practicality of foraging that after reading her book and speaking with her on the phone, I am left wondering why I haven't been eating weeds for years.

Lee grew up hiking and fishing along the banks of the Mississippi with her grandfather and father. They taught her about plant identification, but it wasn't until many years later while gardening in her large organic garden that foraging became part of her life. She described this evolution to me on the phone:

There I was, hoeing and mulching, babying along my vegetables, getting rid of the weeds, and I thought, something is wrong here. Why don't I study these weeds? Could they be useful? I wasn't spraying any chemicals . . . the weeds looked so happy and vibrant. God put them right in my garden, and I began to think that maybe I should pay attention. Why spend all this time getting rid of weeds, when they are the easiest thing to grow and maybe I can use them? I am a practical person.

During nine years of eating wild food every day, Lee allowed herself to trust her own intuition about the nutritional and medicinal qualities of plants, and their safety. She has since learned that many of the conclusions she has drawn about plants are the exact tenets of ancient teachings and are part of the wisdom of Native Americans.

NUTRITIONAL BENEFITS OF WEEDS

From the moment in her garden when Lee really looked at weeds as food, she has been doing research into their nutritional benefits, ultimately leading to a Ph.D. in nutrition. While she studied all the scantily available literature on the subject, her biggest teacher has been her direct experience. "I would go backpacking by myself, taking almost no food, and I discovered that by eating small amounts of wild foods I felt wonderfully energetic, and I didn't need to eat very much. I discovered wild plants are powerhouses of nutrition."

The weeds that are the most nutritious and abundant, Lee says, are in places where the soil has been disturbed, such as a garden.

The weed's role is to come and heal the imbalance of the soil. Clover fixes nitrogen, for example; burdock root is a very deep taproot that will go into soil that has become too compact. Burdock's roots will break up tightly packed soil, and in doing so bring nutrients up from the subsoil. Despite this value, in some states burdock is considered a "noxious weed," even illegal, so the county will come spray it with herbicides, right in the farmer's field, even though it is reaching down to the deep soil to give nutrients to the topsoil. Now you decide which makes more sense, using dangerous chemicals to control a bold invader or understanding that the soil is in trouble and correcting the problem so burdock won't need to do so.

Lee remarks that burdock has some very interesting medicinal properties, as do many of the invasive weeds.

Not only is burdock a blood purifier, but it is also a male potency aid for sexual endurance. Would male farmers kill burdock if they knew that? Would their wives let them?

"The plants are shouting at us, yelling at us, saying 'Here I am,' and yet humans in their arrogance mow them down, and pull them out, stepping away from the observation of the natural cycles," says Lee. She explains that commercial produce (such as broccoli or apples) has been hybridized time after time; produce has been bred for such traits as size, flavor, and resistance to fungus, but not nutrition.

Whenever you breed for one thing, you are going to lose a number of other things, and usually the nutrition is weakened. When I eat a plant that has not been tampered with, I've observed time and time again that all I have to do is eat a little bit of it and I have an incredible amount of energy. I have really lived this. I did it every day for nine years.

Lee believes that wild foods are the ultimate multivitamin pill (if one can make such a sacrilegious comparison!). Whereas commercial vitamins and minerals have been isolated and duplicated by synthetic means, Lee speculates that there is much more value in eating wild plants.

Scientists are realizing that the synergy of ingredients is vital. The blend from the food source itself is so much more than just the vitamins and minerals. Plant food consists of thousands of phytochemicals that all work together as a team. For example, you can't have a symphony with just a cellist, or a football team with just a quarterback. Everything works together in a plant to create a whole. This is why food in capsules are now replacing synthetic vitamin pills. Nature's wild produce is nutrient-dense and synergistically complete.

HOW TO START FORAGING

"Nature is providing a whole abundant grocery store for us, and it's very easy for the gardener or even someone who just goes on a weekend walk or bike ride, to find food," says Lee. She recommends introducing yourself to two or three plants a season, or even a year, so as not to become overwhelmed. To help learn plant identification, Lee advises obtaining a copy of *The Peterson Guide to Edible Plants.* "Identify a plant, nibble on it a little bit, and figure out how to add it to a meal. Try chickweed, lamb's-quarter or violet leaves, for example: they're not much stronger tasting than lettuce."

PRECAUTIONS AND TIPS[†]

1. Know what you are picking. Be sure it is the plant you seek. Many edible plants have a poisonous look-alike.

[†]*Permission to reprint granted by the author, Deborah Lee and Havelin Communications, Inc.*

Once the edible plant has been definitely identified, take a tiny nibble, then wait for thirty minutes to observe any adverse reactions. *Note*: As a general rule of thumb, if a plant has any red or purple on the leaves, leave it alone: 90 percent of the time it will be toxic.

2. Be extremely careful when collecting mushrooms. A novice can easily make mistakes.

3. Know what part to pick. One part of a plant may be safe to eat and another part toxic. For example, elderberry blossoms and fruit are edible, but the leaves and branches are poisonous.

4. Just because wild animals can eat a plant does not mean humans can. Our digestive systems are much different. However, if wildlife are *not* eating a certain tasty-looking morsel, take heed.

5. Avoid plants in commercially fertilized areas. Some plants such as lamb's-quarter absorb toxic levels of nitrates from commercial fertilizer. Also avoid collecting under power lines, in unfamiliar weed lots or lawns, or beside farmers' fields. These areas may be sprayed with herbicides or defoliants to kill the weeds.

6. Avoid foraging close to main roadsides. Plants may be sprayed with toxic weed control chemicals and may be absorbing exhaust from cars.

7. Collect with consciousness. As foragers, we have a responsibility to make the habitat in which we collect a little better for our being there. For example, if you collect dandelion leaves, select three or four from each plant and artistically prune.

8. Take only what you need. Be sure enough plants are left to replenish the supply. Leave some for wildlife. They cannot go to the supermarket.

9. Once the food is collected, clean and sort it in the field or in the woods. No cook wants a sink full of muddy dandelion greens mingled with grass blades and half an anthill!

10. Practice moderation and avoid gorging yourself on wild edibles. They are powerful foods and your system may

need to adjust. Eating them may cause the body to discharge various toxins or impurities. You want this beneficial cleansing to occur slowly.

11. Learn to blend wild produce into a meal. Many wild foods have very strong flavors. To simply boil, steam, or sauté them by themselves may render a rather powerful taste. Chopping a cup of the young leaves and adding them to soup, steaming them with cabbage, or sautéing them with potatoes and onions mellows their flavor.

PUTTING FORAGING INTO PRACTICE

The Seasons

Lee has found that eating wild foods has connected her more to nature. She observes,

I found that when I started to eat wild foods I became more observant of the natural cycles around me. When utilizing wild foods I automatically become more part of the natural process, and start eating with the seasons. Foraging becomes so much fun from season to season. I came to love a particular watercress patch in the spring, when I lived in Pennsylvania, and I looked forward to the hickory nuts in the fall.

The foods available seasonally also provide nourishment appropriate to the body's needs at the different times of year. Lee has found,

In the spring there are more leafy greens, which are very nutritious, light, and uplifting. These foods help us to feel buoyant and help us replenish trace minerals ordinarily lacking in the winter diet. In the summer there are more flowers and eventually fruit. These are things that cool and relax. In the fall and winter there are roots and nuts. Nuts are high in protein and fat, and will last all winter long. Roots are a good source of winter food, they will store well, and are warming, energizing, and high in nutrition . . . exactly what you need.

EXAMPLES OF EDIBLE FOODS TO FORAGE FOR[‡]

Spring Greens: Cattail stalks, dandelion, chickweed, chives, nettles, wild lettuce, violet leaves.

Spring Flowers, Fruits, and Berries: Flowers—Redbud, mustard and rose family, violets. Berries—strawberry, gooseberry.

Spring Roots: Burdock, dandelion, wild parsnip.

Summer Herbs: Clover flowers, horsetail tops, chamomile flowers, raspberry leaves, yarrow, bergamot.

Summer Fruits and Berries: Chokeberries, raspberries, mulberries, wild plum.

Summer Greens: Grape leaves, lamb's-quarter, amaranth, wood sorrel.

Fall Roots, Tubers, and Rhizomes: Daylily, Jerusalem artichoke, marshmallow, burdock, wild parsnip.

Fall Greens: Purslane, watercress, dandelion.

Fall Nuts: Hazelnut, pecan, hickory, acorn, walnut.

Fall Fruits and Berries: Grape, hawthorn, chokeberry, wintergreen, wild apples.

Winter Greens: Chives, garlic mustard, watercress, thistle.

Winter Roots and Tubers: Arrowhead, burdock, cattail, thistle.

Winter Fruits and Berries: Bayberry, juniper berry, wintergreen berry, rose hip.

COLLECTING

Collecting foraged food doesn't need to take a lot of extra time because you can pick the foods when you are gardening or walking. "Whenever I hike I always have a little backpack . . . I get exercise *and* something for supper," says Lee. She emphasizes that starting in the garden is the easiest way to begin. "Chickweed is everywhere in the spring," she enthuses, "just add it to the basket of your harvested vegetables. Eat the weeds, don't curse them. They'll become your friend . . . free food of the healthiest kind. What more can you want?"

[‡]*The above excerpts from charts in* Exploring Nature's Uncultivated Garden *have been printed by permission of the publisher, Havelin Communications, Inc.*

FOOD PACKAGING

Note: For the health and environmental impact of packaging materials, please see chapter 2. For recycling information, please see chapter 6.

No discussion of buying groceries is complete without discussing the fact that shoppers are in the midst of a food packaging nightmare. According to the USDA, for every ten dollars we spend at the grocery store, one dollar goes toward packaging. By the year 2000, 73 percent of landfills will be closed because they are full. Throwing away our food packaging is going to get more and more expensive, both for our pocketbooks and for the environment. And the worst of it is that most of us don't even *want* fancy packaging for our food.

Some of us share a fantasy of going to a supermarket, buying a week's groceries for a family of four, and after going through the checkout line, taking all the packaging off the food and leaving it in a heap (it would be a large one) for the supermarket to dispose of. True, that wouldn't be fair to the supermarket (it isn't entirely their fault), but it would send a message that too much packaging is wasteful and not appreciated.

Believe it or not, it is illegal in Germany to place any packaging in landfills or to burn it in incinerators. German manufacturers, distributors, and retail stores are duty bound to take back all shipping, display, and retail packaging, and either reuse it or recycle it.

SHOPPING WITH AN EYE TO PACKAGING

Every town and city in the country has a different capacity for recycling packaging waste. All discussion here about what kind of packaging to buy is meaningless unless it applies specifically to your community. Knowing your town's recycling system, however, *will* enable you to make educated decisions about what packaging you choose to bring home. Call your town's or city's recycling center. Most have brochures to offer you and clear guidelines for you to follow.

There are some guidelines for buying packaging that apply to all of us. The more you understand the following principles, the less packaging waste you will have for the landfill or incinerator.

REDUCE

Whenever possible, choose food with a minimal amount of packaging. One way to accomplish this is to buy food in bulk, large sizes, or in concentrates.

RECYCLED

Try to buy food packaged with recycled glass, paper, or aluminum. (Recycled plastics are not allowed to be used for food packaging, except for berry baskets, egg cartons, and some soda bottles.) Some manufacturers don't put the recycled icon on the package, so when in doubt call 800 directory assistance and ask for the manufacturer's number.

To determine if the packaging you are buying was made with 100 percent recycled and recyclable materials, look for the recycled icon: three arrows on a black circular background. Three arrows on a white background within a circle is used when only a percentage of recycled materials have been used.

RECYCLABLE

If packaging waste can be collected and recycled in most communities in the country, the Federal Trade Commission declares the package can be labeled recyclable. (Even so, check to see if the packaging is actually recyclable in your community.) If only part of the package is recyclable, that information needs to be clearly stated on the package. Three arrows without any background means that the packaging is recyclable.

REUSABLE

Whenever possible, buy reusable, not disposable, products, such as razors, drinking cups, plates, utensils, and napkins. Also, reuse food packaging, particularly plastic and glass. For example, store leftovers in glass jars or yogurt containers to reduce your consumption of plastic wrap or aluminum foil. But reusing packaging can also be a safety risk, so you need to use good judgment. Some general rules of thumb:

* Only reuse containers that can be washed thoroughly.
* Never reuse containers that have contained chemicals (for cleaning or pest control, for instance).
* To reduce risk of bacteria poisoning, do not reuse any packing that came in contact with meat or dairy products unless thoroughly sterilized.

REFILLABLE

You may be lucky enough to live near a store that sells refillable products—the store will fill plastic and glass containers with such products as honey, laundry detergent, shampoo, and food oils. Health food stores and green supermarkets commonly have refillable products.

PAPER OR PLASTIC GROCERY BAGS?

The best answer to this question we are all asked at the checkout counter of the supermarket is: canvas! Otherwise recycle and reuse; both paper and plastic have advantages and disadvantages. The problem with plastic is that even though the bags can be recycled, only a small number actually are. Some communities do not even have the capacity to recycle plastic bags. Choose plastic only if you can recycle the bags, and then recycle them! Reuse brown paper bags as much as possible before recycling.

4

The Green Pantry

A pantry full of whole grains and flours, nuts and seeds, dry beans and peas, teas and oils, is one of the most important tools for making cooking with whole foods convenient. The foods recommended in this chapter for your pantry are also excellent sources of nutrition, providing fiber, complex carbohydrates, essential fatty acids, crucial minerals such as zinc and iron, and much, much more. The nutritional benefits of these foods cannot be emphasized enough. All you need to add for a well-balanced diet are fresh fruits and vegetables, and dairy and other animal products if you choose. Pantry foods are also very versatile and can be used to make delicious, flavorful meals.

The history of how different grains, nuts, dried beans, and herbs and spices fanned out across the world is fascinating, as it follows the travels of the global explorers and the meanderings of the spice and silk trades. Soybeans and adzuki beans came from China, lentils from the Mediterranean; black-eyed peas became popular in Africa after being imported from China, chickpeas came from India, and black, pinto, and red kidney beans came from the Americas. Cookbooks of the world's foods are gold mines of information about interesting and flavorful ways of using these global staples.

Even though most of the foods recommended for your pantry originated in foreign lands, almost all are now grown in the United States. Whenever possible, buy U.S. grown. Shipping foods more or less halfway around the world takes a high environmental toll. Try to track down the sources of your food and find alternatives to those that are imported. Buying pecans grown along the Mississippi for a snack, instead of macadamias grown in Australia, for example, makes good environmental sense. Each pantry category that follows contains a glossary that will introduce you to the varieties of foods cultivated in the United States.

GRAINS AND FLOURS

Cereal grains are the fruits of the grass family. Wheat, rye, barley, oats, corn, millet, and rice are all true cereals. Some seeds and berries—buckwheat, for example—are treated as grains although in fact they are not from the grass family. A typical grain kernel is made up of a hull or husk, which protects the whole; bran, which holds the kernel together; the germ or embryo, which is the grain's seed and contains about 90 percent of the nutritional content of the kernel; and the endosperm, which is mostly starch. Grain kernels are steel-cut, rolled, flaked, and ground into meals and flours.

Whole grains are some of our most important sources of complex carbohydrates, starch, and fiber. Many grains, such as oats, contain components that help the body reduce high serum cholesterol levels. The soluble fiber in whole grains can help reduce insulin elevations after eating. Whole grains are a main staple in the diet for people all over the world.

Most flours are derived from a whole cereal grain that has been milled into a fine meal and is then used for making baked goods of all kinds. Modern milling of whole cereal grains puts the kernel through a high-heat milling process that removes the germ and bran, leaving only the endosperm (starch). The endosperm is then ground into different sizes for different purposes. The result is a "refined" flour. Refined wheat flour is often bleached with chlorine dioxide to make it white, and it is chemically aged with potassium bromate or iodate to improve its baking properties. It is then "enriched" by adding some but not all of the vitamins that were stripped from the grain during the milling process.

The stone-ground milling process is the most popular method of milling that does not remove the bran or germ, and the result is a whole grain flour. Mills that produce stone-ground grains exist all across the United States; some are old and still powered by water, and others new and run by electricity. Flours from mills that stone grind are commonly available in health food stores, specialty mail-order catalogs, and green supermarkets. Stone-ground flours are usually marked as such.

The nutritional comparison of refined white flour and whole wheat flour is striking and is a convincing reason to switch to whole grains from refined. Many of the nutrients eliminated in the grinding process in refined grains, such as vitamin E, are crucial to good health. Refined wheat flour is so nutritionally insufficient farmers report that even bugs die when trying to sustain themselves on it in silos.

If you think about it, the primary ingredients of refined foods—donuts, cakes, white bread, crackers, cereal—which make them refined are "white" flour and sugar. If you replace the refined white flour with a whole grain flour at every opportunity, you can virtually eliminate refined foods from your diet (barring the occasional sugary dessert). Cereals, pastas, and breads all have a whole grain alternative. And by choosing whole grains instead of refined, the flavor and nutritional value of the food is substantially improved. "The closer I stay to using only flour from whole grain grown in simple, organic partnership with the environment, the better my breads taste and look," writes Daniel Leader in his book *Bread Alone*.

Replacing refined grains with whole grains does not mean having to eat food that is too heavy. Softer whole grains such as barley, oat, millet, teff, and brown rice grind into flours that are light in texture and color and have mellow, mild flavors. They can easily be substituted at any time for white flour. Even pastas can be made successfully with whole grain flours; one is not limited to chewy, dense whole wheat spaghetti if one wants to provide a whole grain pasta dish. Brown rice noodles are light-flavored and slightly nutty tasting, for example; they are fine textured and look virtually identical to "normal" spaghetti.

There are many delicious grains and flours, both familiar and unfamiliar, to experiment with during the process of trying to make one's diet more wholesome: quinoa, buckwheat, barley, kamut, rice, spelt, teff, oats, and triticale. Ancient grains such as quinoa are gaining widespread popularity due to their high protein and nutrient content and appealing taste.

Freshness and Storage

Millers of the early twentieth century were delighted with the new, high-heat milling process that removed both bran and germ; the germ (full of oil rich in vitamin E) no longer gummed up the grinding mill, and without the oil the flour's shelf life became infinitely longer. Unlike refined flours, whole grain flours do not have a long shelf life. It is the oil itself, found in the germ, that becomes rancid. Either whole grain flours should be ground right before use (the ideal solution) or bought in small quantities at a time and stored in the refrigerator or freezer—like perishable fruits and vegetables—until use. Unrefined flours should not be stored for longer than a month! They should be stored in a cool, dry, dark cupboard. Ideally, unrefined flours should be stored in a refrigerator or freezer, where they will last a bit longer. Refined flours should be kept no more than six months.

Small, manual flour mills are available for around $60. Small electric flour mills that grind with stone cost around $250. (See chapter 6.) Grinding your own flours does not take much effort and will provide you with high-quality flours rich in flavor and nutrition. Health food stores rarely have grain mills to use on the premises, but there is no harm in asking.

Unhulled grains can last for centuries. The hull completely protects the oils from rancidity. Before cooking, grains in their hull need to be soaked to soften the hull, which will speed along the cooking. Always rinse grains thoroughly before using.

Weevils, sometimes called cereal moths, can be pests in the warmer months. They settle into boxes of cereal, rice, and other grain storage bins. The best way to deter weevils is to place bay leaves in the storage bins, boxes, or jars. Weevils hate the smell and will vacate the area. Fortunately, the grains do not absorb the flavor of the herb.

Cooking Grains

WHOLE GRAINS

A good electric grain steamer (commonly called a rice steamer) is a very useful tool to help you cook whole grains with little difficulty. You can make a hot cereal from whole grain porridge for breakfast, or flavorful side dishes, cold salads, and additions to soups and stews. Follow manufacturers' directions for steaming times. In general, use one-quarter to one-half cup less liquid for electric steamers than is called for in stove-top cooking. For more on recommended steaming equipment, see chapter 6.

To cook whole grains in a regular pot on a stove, bring the required amount of water to a boil (see table on page 126), stir in the grain, return the water to a boil, cover, lower the heat, and cook until the liquid is absorbed. If the grain is not tender, or the liquid is not absorbed, cover and cook for a few minutes longer.

GUIDE TO GRAINS AND FLOURS

AMARANTH

A small seed, about the size of a poppy seed; not actually a grain.

> Gluten: No
> Origin: The Americas
> Current Cultivation: Asia, Africa, the Americas
> Protein Benefit: Unusually high amino acid lysine content makes it an excellent protein

Whole Amaranth

Breakfast cereal (needs to be boiled), "popcorn" (use amaranth seeds instead of popcorn), side dishes like rice, salads. Because amaranth is sticky and glutinous, a good rule of thumb is to use it in a one-to-three ratio with other grains.

Cooking Times for Whole Grains

Grain (1 cup)	Water (cups)	Cooking Time (mins.)	Yield (in cups)
Amaranth	3	25	2½
Barley, flakes	2	15–20	2½
Barley, pearled	3	60	3½
Barley, whole soaked	3	120–180	3½
Buckwheat groats/kasha	2	15–20	3
Cornmeal	4	20–25	3
Hominy grits	4	25	3½
Kamut flakes	2	15	2½
Kamut groats	3	35–45	3½
Millet	2½ to 3	30–40	3½
Oat groats	4	60	3
Oats/rolled	1½	10	2½
Oats/steel-cut	4	40–45	3
Polenta	1	15	2½
Quinoa	2	15	3½
Rice, basmati	2	45	3
Rice, brown	2 to 2½	45–50	3–4
Rice, long-grain	2	15	3–4
Rice, medium-/short-grain	1¾	15	3
Rice, parboiled	2 to 2½	20–25	3–4
Rye, berries	3½	60	3
Rye, cracked	3	45	3
Rye, flaked	2	20	2½
Sorghum, whole	2 to 2½	45–50	3
Teff, whole	3	15	3
Triticale, berries	3½	60	2½
Triticale, flakes	2	20	2½
Wheat, berries	3½	60	2½
Wheat, bulgur	2	30	2½
Wheat, couscous	2	15	3
Wheat, cracked	3	20	2½
Wheat, flakes	2	15	2½
Wild rice	2½	40	3

Amaranth Flour

Substitute equally, but don't use much more than ¼ cup.

ARROWROOT

The starch of the maranta root. Not a grain; used as a grain substitute.

Gluten: No
Origin: The tropics
Current Cultivation: Caribbean

Ground/powdered Arrowroot

A thickener; substitute equally for cornstarch. Can be used in desserts; it is very fine, very similar to cornstarch. To substitute for a flour thickener, use 1 tablespoon arrowroot for every 2½ tablespoons all-purpose flour.

BARLEY

A cereal grain with a nutty flavor.

Gluten: Yes, low amounts
Origin: North Africa, China, Mediterranean
U.S. Cultivation: Yes

Whole Barley

The most nutritious way of using barley, as only the husk is removed. Cold salad, bread, baked goods, pilaf, hot cereal.

Cooking Tip: Needs to be cooked for a while to become chewy. Soak the grain overnight to reduce cooking time. Cook until chewy.

Barley Flour

The flour is light-tasting, resembling refined white flour in this way and therefore makes excellent quick breads, muffins, and scones. Because it contains small amounts of gluten it should be combined with a higher gluten flour for yeast breads.

Substitution: To substitute for all-purpose flour, use ¾ of the amount of barley flour.

Pearl Barley

A more refined barley. Used in soups, casseroles, salads.

Cooking Directions: Steam with broth for casseroles and salads, simmer in the soup for an hour.

Barley Flakes

Made from pearl barley, barley flakes can be made into a hot cereal or added to breads.

Cooking Directions: For cereal, cook in a ratio of one part barley flakes to one part water. For other purposes, use as you would oats.

BUCKWHEAT/KASHA

A seed; not in the wheat family. Roasted buckwheat groats are dark brown and are commonly called kasha; white buckwheat (unroasted) is very hard to find but has a blander flavor. Chemicals are not needed to grow buckwheat, as the plants are naturally pest resistant.

Gluten: Yes, very small amount
Origin: Russia
U.S. Cultivation: Yes
Protein Benefit: Provides all eight amino acids

Whole Buckwheat

Called kasha, it is commonly used in pilafs, breads, and any way one would use rice.

Cooking Tip: Coat the groats in a raw egg (one egg for each cup of groats) and then roast in a pan for three minutes. This technique is used to protect the seed from absorbing too much water so the kasha won't get mushy.

Buckwheat Flour

A dark brown flour made from roasted buckwheat, it is strong flavored, and used primarily in pancakes and muffins.

Soba Noodles

Japanese noodles made of roasted buckwheat and wheat.

Udon Noodles

Japanese noodles made from unroasted buckwheat and wheat.

BULGUR

See Wheat.

CHICKPEA FLOUR/GRAHAM FLOUR/BESAN FLOUR

Made from ground, unroasted chickpeas.

> Gluten: No
> Origin: Middle East
> U.S. Cultivation: Yes
> Protein Benefit: Very high protein
> Uses: Dishes such as falafel, Indian fritters; thickener

> *Cooking Tip:* For breads—both yeast and quick—substitute ¼ cup chickpea flour for each cup of wheat flour.

CORN/MAIZE

Corn is eaten in many different ways, from corn bread to corn on the cob to popcorn. A cereal grain, it grows in many colors, from yellow to rust to blue-black.

> Gluten: No
> Origin: The Americas
> U.S. Cultivation: Yes

Cornmeal

Usually mixed half and half with refined wheat flour for corn bread; try experimenting with using all cornmeal or substituting brown rice, barley, or millet flour for the refined white wheat flour. Excellent for making quick breads.

Blue Cornmeal

Use as per cornmeal. Also excellent for tortillas.

Polenta

Finely ground Italian cornmeal that is cooked to resemble cream of wheat and often served baked, as a side dish.

Hominy

The corn kernel's hull is removed, and the kernel dried. To cook hominy it needs to be soaked (in milk, if you want) for eight hours or so, and then cooked at a low heat for many (three to five) hours. Added to casseroles and baked.

Grits

Ground hominy. Cook to the consistency of a mushy hot cereal, served as a side dish.

Masa Harina

Also a form of ground hominy, masa harina is used to make tortillas and corn chips.

Popcorn

Whole corn kernels are heated in a covered pan until the kernels explode into white, fluffy balls about five times the size of the kernel.

Corn Pastas

One hundred percent corn noodles are available in most health food stores.

DURUM SEMOLINA

See Wheat.

KAMUT

Traced back to around 4000 B.C., kamut is an "ancient" cereal grain that is being repopularized because of its rich, buttery flavor. Kamut is related to wheat, though kamut is completely natural, having never been hybrid.

  Gluten: Yes
  Origin: North Africa, the Middle East
  U.S. Cultivation: Yes, first introduced in 1989

Whole Kamut

Whole kamut will cook faster if soaked for many hours. Eat as hot cereal, side dish, grain salad.

Kamut Flour

As a whole grain flour, kamut flour is lighter than whole wheat. Excellent for muffins, breads; all wheat-based recipes.

  Flour Substitute: Substitute 2½ cups of kamut flour for 2 cups of white wheat flour.

Kamut Flakes

Use just as you would oatmeal.

Kamut Pastas

Available in health food stores.

MILLET

A true cereal grain, millet is a small seed and is related to sorghum.

Gluten: No
Origin: Africa, Asia
U.S. Cultivation: Yes

Whole Millet

Excellent addition to soups and stews, breakfast cereal, and side dish.

Millet Flour

Works very well for quick breads such as muffins.

Millet Flakes

Use just as you would oatmeal.

OATS

A true cereal grain.

Gluten: Yes
Origin: Asia, Middle East
U.S. Cultivation: Yes

Oat Groats

The kernel with the hull removed (but the germ and bran are still intact). Used as a side dish and in pilafs.

Steel-Cut Oats

Cut groats. Delicious as a hot cereal and in other baked goods such as breads and cookies.

Rolled Oats

Cut groats that are steamed to soften and then rolled into flakes. Use as you would steel-cut oats.

Quick Oats

Like rolled oats, except the cut is finer. While less flavorful, quick oats can make a good hot cereal on the run.

Instant Oats

The finest cut of the oat; the resulting hot cereal is very mushy and much less flavorful than less fine "cuts" of the groat.

Oat Bran

Not a whole food, as the germ and endosperm are removed from the oat kernel.

POTATO FLOUR

The starch from potatoes, this flour is used as a thickener but also as a flour substitute in gluten-free diets.

Gluten: No
Origin: South America

Substitution: A flavorless powder, it can be substituted equally for cornstarch for thickening, or, for a baked dish, substitute ⅝ cup potato flour for one cup white flour.

QUINOA

Related to buckwheat and amaranth, quinoa is a round seed the size of a sesame seed. Increasingly popular because it is high in protein and has a quick cooking time and mild flavor. Sometimes called the "vegetarian caviar."

Gluten: No
Origin: South America
U.S. Cultivation: Yes
Protein Benefit: Complete amino acid balance

Whole Quinoa

Hot cereal, salads, side dishes, served like rice.

Cooking Tip: Wash carefully before cooking to remove saponin coating, which can be bitter. Rinse and drain five times or more.

Storage Tip: Quinoa has a very short shelf life due to its oil content. Buy a small amount at a time.

RICE

An aquatic cereal grain and a main staple of the diet in much of the world.

> Gluten: No
> Origin: Southeast Asia
> U.S. Cultivation: Yes
> Uses: Used in everything from casseroles to side dishes to cold salads
> The following are U.S.-grown rice products.

Arborio
Used to make risotto; available in white and brown varieties.

Basmati
Traditionally grown in Pakistan and India and aged for one year, it is an aromatic rice that is also grown in the United States.

Brown Rice
The least processed form of rice. The outer hull is removed, but not the bran.

Della
An aromatic rice similar to basmati.

Jasmine
An aromatic rice; stickier than basmati or della. (Ninety percent of the jasmine rice available in this country is imported.)

Long-, Medium-, or Short-Grain Rice

Refers to its length in relationship to its width. Long-grain rice is four to five times as long as it is wide, for example. There is no nutritional difference among rices of different lengths.

Parboiled or Converted Rice

Rice that is soaked, steamed, and dried before milling. More nutritious than regular-milled white rice.

Rice Bran

The bran and germ of the rice grain. This is not a whole food. It is added to cereals, muffins, and other baked goods.

Rice Flour

Look for brown rice flour. A very delicate flour, brown rice flour makes delicious baked goods such as muffins and cookies.

   Substitute: Substitute ⅞ cup rice flour for one cup all-purpose flour.

Texamati

Similar to the aromatic basmati, it is actually a crossbreed of basmati and long-grain rice. Grown in Texas. Available as brown rice or refined white.

Wehani

A basmati hybrid, it has a reddish color.

White Rice

Also referred to as "polished"; the hull, bran, and most of the germ is removed in the milling process (refined).

Wild Rice

See Wild Rice, page 141.

Rice Storage

Cooked rice can stay in the refrigerator up to one week, tightly covered, or frozen up to six months. Uncooked brown rice has a shelf life of about six months. To reheat cooked rice, add two tablespoons of water or broth for each cup of rice. Cover and cook on low for five minutes.

RYE

A cereal grain, the strong-flavored rye is widely used mixed with wheat in breads.

> Gluten: Yes, low amounts
> Origin: Southwest Asia
> U.S. Cultivation: Yes
> Uses: Bread; rye berries: side dishes such as pilaf

Rye Berries

Side dishes, casseroles, cold salads.

Rye Flour

The darker the flour, the more bran has been retained during the milling process. Pumpernickel is the least refined of the rye flours.
> *Flour Substitute:* Substitute 1¼ cups rye flour for 1 cup white flour.

Cracked Rye

Coarse meal.

Rye Flakes

Cereal like oatmeal.

SORGHUM

Related to millet; the seeds are similar.

> Gluten: No
> Origin: Africa, Asia
> U.S. Cultivation: Yes

Whole Sorghum

Use as you would rice or millet; used in Africa for flat unleavened bread.

SOY FLOUR

High-protein flour made from soybeans.

> Gluten: No
> Origin: Asia
> U.S. Cultivation: Yes
> Uses: Substitute up to ¼ cup soy flour for ¼ cup white flour

SPELT

Related to wheat, but unlike wheat, spelt has not been hybridized.

> Gluten: Yes
> Origin: Middle East
> U.S. Cultivation: Yes

Spelt Berries

Use as a side dish as you would rice.

Spelt Flakes

Follow the directions for oatmeal.

Spelt Flour

Substitute for wheat equally.

TAPIOCA

Starch from a tropical root. Used as a grain substitute.

> Gluten: No
> Origin: The tropics

Pearl Tapioca

Famous for making tapioca pudding.

Tapioca Flour

Substitute for cornstarch or arrowroot.

Cooking Tip: As a thickener, substitute 1½ tablespoons tapioca flour for 1 tablespoon white flour.

TEFF

A tiny red, brown, or white seed. White teff is the mildest.

> Gluten: No
> Origin: Africa
> U.S. Cultivation: Yes

Whole Teff

Great for hot cereal and as a change from rice.

Teff Flour

Most commonly made into Ethiopian *injera* bread, teff flour is mild in flavor and light-textured.

TRITICALE

A hybrid cereal grain, cross between wheat and rye; more nutritious than either wheat or rye.

> Gluten: Yes
> Origin: 1937 hybrid
> U.S. Cultivation: Yes

Triticale Berries

Breakfast cereal, side dishes.

Triticale Flakes

Follow directions for oatmeal.

Triticale Flour

Substitute equally for wheat or rye flour.

WHEAT

A cereal grain, wheat is the main grain staple in the American diet.

> Gluten: Yes
> Origin: Middle East
> U.S. Cultivation: Yes

Wheat Berries

Wheat kernels.

Bulgur

Wheat kernel is steamed, dried, ground.

Wheat Flakes

Whole wheat kernels that have been cut.

Couscous

Made from durum semolina, the bran and germ are missing.

Cracked Wheat

Whole wheat kernels dried and cracked (not cooked) between rollers.

Farina

Finely ground cracked wheat.

Durum

Hard wheat; higher gluten content than soft wheat.

Seitan

Often used as a meat substitute; the bran is rinsed away, leaving the gluten, which is kneaded until it has a meatlike texture. Not a whole food, but it is high in protein.

Soft Wheat

Low-gluten wheat.

Flour

All-Purpose/White Flour

Refined wheat flour; the germ and bran have been removed during milling. All-purpose flour turns white naturally with age, but some all-purpose flour has been bleached and bromated.

Whole Wheat Flour

Flour that has been milled in a way that retains the bran and the germ. Much darker in color than white flour, it is more flavorful than white flour, with a denser and heavier texture.

Bread Flour

Made from high-gluten refined hard wheat.

Graham Flour

A whole grain flour.

Pastry/Cake Flour

Refined white flour; made from low-gluten soft wheat.

Semolina

Made from durum wheat; the bran and germ are removed from flour during milling, unless the label states "100 percent unrefined durum semolina."

Pastas

Most pastas are made from semolina, a refined durum wheat. You can be assured that the pasta is made out of a whole grain only if the label states "whole durum wheat semolina." Most pastas have been enriched.

WILD RICE

An aquatic grass seed grain that has been hand-picked in the wild.

Origin: North America

U.S. Cultivation: Exclusive to North America; hand cultivated

Uses: Very expensive; added to rice dishes for flavor and texture

See the appendix for the nutritional contents of grains and other whole foods.

DRIED BEANS AND PEAS

Dried beans are extremely versatile. Added herbs and spices can transform them into everything from the Middle Eastern dish hummus, to black bean soup, to Mexican tacos. Beans are not complete proteins (the only exception being the soybean) because they lack one or more of the essential amino acids, yet according to some nutritionists they become perfect proteins, even better than those of animal products, when combined with whole grains, nuts, seeds, or animal products.

Beans are a superb source of protein, complex carbohydrates, and soluble fiber and have only a small percentage of fat, if any, and no cholesterol. They are rich in vitamins and minerals, particularly calcium and iron. According to nutritionists, beans are excellent foods for diabetics, hypoglycemics, and those with insulin resistance because components found in beans do not trigger the over-release of insulin, which can be translated in the body into fat.

Dried beans are in fact legumes. They are the dried seeds from pods of plants. There are approximately thirteen thousand species of beans, from six hundred genera. While we only discuss ten in the glossary below, more and more species are finding their way into specialty stores. Called "boutique" beans, some are derived from hybrids and others from heirloom seeds (see chapter 2). Some of the more unusual of these include anasazi, appaloosa, black runner, black valentine, calypso, cranberry, Florida butter, Jackson wonder, pigeon, rattlesnake, scarlet runner, specked lima, winged and wren's egg. Buying or growing unusual beans from heirloom seeds is an excellent way of protecting biodiversity.

Cooking Beans

SOAKING

As a rule of thumb, use two to three cups of water for each cup of beans.

Soaking Overnight

All dried beans except lentils and peas need to be soaked for many hours—ideally overnight—to soften them before cooking. Before soaking, make sure to wash the beans thoroughly to remove any stones or dirt that may have lodged in them. When soaking is complete, make sure to rinse the beans thoroughly.

Quick-Soak Method

If you forget to soak beans overnight, there is a quick way of soaking beans that works very well. Soak the beans for as long as you can, rinse, and then place in a pot and cover with water. Bring the beans to a rapid boil for a few minutes, remove from the heat, cover, and let sit for an hour. Rinse the beans thoroughly (for the same reason mentioned above), replace the water with clean water, and proceed with the recipe. If soaked for a few hours before the quick boil, beans generally need only about half an hour of actual cooking time to reach the right texture and softness for eating.

PRESSURE COOKER METHOD

Another method of cooking beans that saves considerable time is using a pressure cooker. Beans can be cooked in a pressure cooker in just fifteen or twenty minutes.

TIPS

* Increase cooking and soaking time in hard water and high-altitude areas.

* Add ⅛ teaspoon baking soda to the pot if you have hard water.
* Salt can halt the process of softening, so do not add until the very end.
* Acids slow the softening of beans. Add acid-based foods such as tomatoes and vinegar as late in the cooking process as possible.
* The Mexicans cook their beans with the herb epazote to reduce flatulence.

Coriander, cumin, and ginger reportedly also reduce flatulence.

SUBSTITUTING CANNED BEANS FOR FRESH

The flavor of canned beans isn't as fresh and flavorful as home-soaked and cooked, nor is there as rich a variety available. However, having some canned beans in your pantry for a quick dinner can be convenient.

The general rule of thumb is one pound of soaked and cooked beans equals approximately five to six cups. When using canned,

Soaking and Cooking Times for Beans
(in hours)

	Soaking Time	Cooking Time	Pressure Cooker
Adzuki	4	1–2	15
Black beans	4	1–2	15
Black-eyed peas	none	1	10
Cannellini beans	4	1–2	15
Chickpeas	4	2–3	25
Lentils	none	½–1	12
Navy	4	1–2	15
Pinto	4	1–2	20
Kidney	4	1	20
Soybeans	12	3–4	30

substitute two to three fifteen-ounce or sixteen-ounce cans of beans for a pound of cooked beans. Each can of beans measures about one and three-quarters to two cups.

STORAGE

Dried beans should be kept in tightly covered containers in a dry place. Cooked beans can be frozen for four to six months, or kept in the refrigerator for four to five days. For best results, freeze beans as a prepared dish.

GUIDE TO BASIC BEANS

ADZUKI

Small brown beans with white keel.

> Origin: Asia
> U.S. Cultivated: Yes
> Fat and Fiber per ½ Cup Cooked: Zero grams fat; seven grams fiber
> Uses: Commonly sprouted; excellent for salads and sweet dishes

BLACK BEANS

Black kidney-shaped beans with a white keel.

> Origin: South America
> U.S. Cultivated: Yes
> Fat and Fiber per ½ Cup Cooked: Zero grams fat; seven grams fiber
> Uses: Many Mexican, South American, Spanish, Cuban dishes; soups, casseroles

BLACK-EYED PEAS

Cream-colored bean with an oval black keel.

Origin: Asia

U.S. Cultivated: Yes

Fat and Fiber per ½ Cup Cooked: Zero grams fat; six grams fiber

Uses: African dishes; brought to America by the slaves and became part of plantation cooking

CANNELLINI BEANS/GREAT NORTHERN BEANS

Long thin white beans.

Origin: South America

U.S. Cultivation: Yes

Fat and Fiber per ½ Cup Cooked: Zero grams fat; six grams fiber

Uses: Italian dishes, pastas, salads, soups, stews, Boston baked beans

CHICKPEAS/GARBANZO BEANS

Round, tan beans about ¼ inch wide.

Origin: Africa, Middle East

U.S. Cultivated: Yes

Fat and Fiber per ½ Cup Cooked: Two grams fat; five grams fiber

Uses: Famous for the Middle Eastern dishes falafel and hummus; also good for salads and stews

KIDNEY BEANS

Maroon beans shaped like kidneys, about half an inch long.

Origin: Asia

U.S. Cultivated: Yes

Fat and Fiber per ½ Cup Cooked: Zero grams fat; six grams fiber

Uses: Chilis, stews, salads

LENTILS

Round, thin beans that are red, yellow, green, or brown.

Origin: Asia
U.S. Cultivated: Yes
Fat and Fiber per ½ Cup Cooked: Zero grams fat; six to eight grams fiber
Uses: Dals, soups, stews

NAVY BEANS

A white bean similar to the cannellini bean.

Origin: Asia
U.S. Cultivation: Yes
Fat and Fiber per ½ Cup Cooked: One-half gram fat; eight grams fiber
Uses: Soups, stews, salads

PINTO BEANS

Brown speckled tan beans about half an inch long.

Origin: Asia, the Americas
U.S. Cultivated: Yes
Fat and Fiber per ½ Cup Cooked: Zero grams fat; seven grams fiber
Uses: Chilis, stews, salads, tacos

SOYBEANS

Small tan round beans about a quarter inch round. Black soybeans are used in Chinese black bean sauces.

Origin: Asia
U.S. Cultivation: Yes
Fat and Fiber per ½ Cup Cooked: Eight grams fat; five grams fiber
Uses: Bean curd (tofu), stir-fry dishes, salads, stews

NUTS AND SEEDS

In a six-year study of twenty-six thousand Seventh-Day Adventists, those participants who consumed nuts at least five times a week had only half the rate of heart attacks or coronary death as those who ate them rarely, and those who ate nuts twice a week had 25 percent less chance of heart disease than those who never ate nuts. The participants who ate nuts were also significantly thinner.

In a five-year study of thirty-four thousand women in Iowa, those who ate nuts were 40 percent less likely to die from heart disease than those who never ate them.

With the intense scrutiny that high-fat foods have been getting, nuts and seeds (which are high in fat) have been increasingly relegated to the list of foods one should never eat. But there is a lot about nuts that is worthy of attention, including the intriguing studies, mentioned above, that point to a component in nuts that seems to help prevent heart disease. Nuts and seeds are also rich in minerals. They are excellent additions to the vegetarian diet because of their high zinc and iron content, minerals that exist in low quantities in plant foods. Next to sea vegetables, nuts and seeds have some of the highest mineral content of any of the plant foods.

Nuts and seeds are classified on the USDA's Food Guide Pyramid as protein sources, and other than legumes, they are the only proteins that contain fiber. (*Note:* However, nuts and seeds are not complete proteins and need to be combined with a grain or animal product.) Nuts and seeds are a rich source of essential fatty acids, oils we need in order to survive and be healthy. Most nuts and seeds are high in monounsaturated and polyunsaturated fats, very low in saturated fats, and cholesterol free.

Be this as it may, nuts and seeds are still very high in fat. Chestnuts are the least fatty, with 13 percent of calories from fat, whereas coconuts and macadamia nuts have respectively 88 percent and 95 percent of their calories from fat. For more on fats, see chapter 2.

Nuts that are imported are expensive for the environment. Brazil nuts only grow in the wilds of Brazil, for example, and need to be harvested and shipped many thousands of miles to find their way into your kitchen. Green pumpkin seeds and cashews, also, are only available from overseas. But there are many nuts growing in abundance in the United States: almonds, filberts, sunflower seeds, pecans, peanuts, walnuts, and chestnuts. Nuts such as acorns, butternuts, and walnuts are also excellent foods to forage for.

How to Buy Nuts

Make sure nuts are fresh, and avoid any that are discolored, shriveled, rubbery, obviously moldy, or taste stale. If you buy nuts in bulk, ask the store for permission to taste a sample before buying in quantity. It is the fat in nuts that goes rancid.

* Buy organic nuts when possible, since high-fat foods (like nuts) will have greater concentrations of pesticides.
* Avoid blanched nuts because chemicals may have been used to "blanch" them.
* Buy nuts in the shell because they are the freshest.
* Buy nuts in the fall during their harvest and freeze them.

Storage

General Guidelines

* Nuts in the shell keep the longest—six months to one year.
* Store shelled nuts in the refrigerator in an airtight glass jar for two to three months, a few months longer in the freezer.
* Whole shelled nuts will stay fresher than broken bits.
* When the oils in nuts go rancid the nuts should not be eaten.
* Light makes free radicals in oils. Store nuts in a dark place.

Nut Butters

Freshly ground nut butters are incomparable in flavor to those from jars. For freshness, your best choice is to buy nut butters in a store that will grind them on the spot. Or, if you can, grind your own at home, using a food processor (works well for walnuts) or grinder.

When buying commercial nut butters, avoid partially hydrogenated oils.

Unopened nut butters have a shelf life of six to nine months. The cooler the temperature, the longer the shelf life. Opened nut butters should last for two weeks and need to be stored in the refrigerator.

GUIDE TO NUTS AND SEEDS

ALMOND (SWEET)

A flavorful nut grown widely in California.

Origin: Mediterranean
Current U.S. Cultivation: Yes
Amount Fat Per ⅓ Cup: Nineteen grams; two grams saturated

BRAZIL NUT

Only grows in the wilds along the Amazon River in South America.

Origin: South America
Current U.S. Cultivation: No
Amount Fat Per ⅓ Cup: Thirty-one grams; seven grams saturated

CASHEW

Imported from India and Brazil.

Origin: Brazil
Current U.S. Cultivation: No
Amount Fat Per ⅓ Cup: Twenty-one grams; four grams saturated

CHESTNUT

North America had a chestnut species of its own until a blight destroyed all the trees in the early part of the twentieth century.

Since that time all the chestnut trees are crossbreeds of Asian species.

Cooking Tip: Boil fresh chestnuts for ten minutes, peel, and use in recipes.

Origin: North America, China, Japan, Europe
Current U.S. Cultivation: Yes
Amount Fat Per ⅓ Cup: One-half gram; zero grams saturated

COCONUT

Large hairy shells about five or six inches long.

Origin: Tropics
Currently U.S. Grown: Yes
Amount Fat Per ⅓ Cup: Seventeen grams; fifteen grams saturated

FILBERT (HAZELNUT)

Commonly sold in the shell; small squarish nut with a hearty flavor.

Origin: Europe
Currently U.S. Grown: Yes
Amount Fat Per ⅓ Cup: Twenty-eight grams; two grams saturated

FLAXSEEDS

Small seeds that resemble apple seeds, flaxseeds are pressed to become linseed oil, one of the richest sources of omega-3 oil.

Origin: Europe
U.S. Cultivation: Yes

MACADAMIA NUT

A soft, round, buttery nut.

Origin: Australia
Currently U.S. Grown: Yes
Amount Fat Per ⅓ Cup: Thirty-three grams; five grams saturated

PEANUT

Not technically a nut, but a pea.

> Origin: Brazil
> Currently U.S. Grown: Yes
> Amount Fat Per ⅓ Cup: Twenty-four grams; 3.5 grams saturated
> Uses: Nut butter, snacks, baked goods

Caution: Aflatoxin is a highly carcinogenic mold that grows on peanuts. The Valencia peanut is grown in a drier climate than other peanuts, such as the Runners, and is therefore less likely to have aflatoxin contamination.

PECAN

Native to the United States, pecans have a rich, buttery flavor.

> Origin: North America, the Mississippi River valley
> Currently U.S. Grown: Yes
> Amount Fat Per ⅓ Cup: Twenty-four grams; two grams saturated
> Uses: Baked goods, snacks

Note: Buy pecans in dull brown shells; if they are reddish and shiny they have been dyed.

PINE NUT

The buttery-tasting seeds of pinecones.

> Origin: North America, Southern Europe, Asia
> Currently U.S. Grown: Yes
> Amount Fat Per ⅓ Cup: Twenty-four grams; four grams saturated
> Uses: Italian pesto, snacks, casseroles

PISTACHIO

Light green nut.

> Origin: Mediterranean, Asia

Currently U.S. Grown: Yes
Amount Fat Per ⅓ Cup: Twenty grams; 2.5 grams saturated
Uses: Baked goods, ice creams, snacks

Note: Health food stores do not sell pistachios that have been dyed white or red.

PUMPKIN, SQUASH SEEDS (THE GREEN VARIETY IS CALLED PEPITA)

Thin seeds about half an inch long. Each pumpkin has a hundred or more seeds.

Origin: The Americas
Currently U.S. Grown: Yes
Amount Fat Per ⅓ Cup: Four grams; one gram saturated
Uses: Snacks, baked goods, desserts

SESAME SEEDS

Small tan seeds; quite bland in flavor unless roasted.

Origin: Mediterranean, Asia
Currently U.S. Grown: Yes
Amount Fat Per ⅓ Cup: Twenty-four grams; 3.5 grams saturated
Uses: Many Indian and Mediterranean dishes, breads, desserts

SUNFLOWER SEEDS

Each sunflower has a hundred or more seeds. Each seed is about a quarter of an inch long.

Origin: North America
Currently U.S. Grown: Yes
Amount Fat Per ⅓ Cup: Twenty-four grams; 2.5 grams saturated

WALNUT

A mild, buttery-flavored nut.

Origin: North America, Asia
Currently U.S. Grown: Yes; wild in the Northeast

Amount Fat Per ⅓ Cup: Twenty grams; two grams saturated
Uses. Snacks, baked goods, main and side dishes

Note: The process of shelling walnuts can expose the meat to a
number of different chemicals. Ideally you should buy nuts in their
shell and remove the shells yourself when you are ready to use the
nuts.

HERBS AND SPICES

From spicy salsas and pestos to winter minestrone, herbs and
spices will help bring the grains and beans from your pantry to life.
With their rich diversity of flavors, they will enable you to make a
wide array of ethnic dishes from around the world. One night have
a meal of earthy flavored black bean enchiladas with chilis, another
a tomato-based pasta with basil and oregano, and a third an East
African paprika-based stew with lentils. All of these meals can be
provided from a full pantry; all you need to add are seasonal fruits
and vegetables.

Most herbs and spices are now grown in the United States. But
if a spice such as cardamom has to be imported, even those who
believe most staunchly that one should only eat food grown in one's
local bioregion agree that the environmental cost of transporting
spices is very low because they are light and a minuscule amount is
needed for most households. This is good news, as it would be sad
indeed to give up cinnamon when baking a pumpkin pie, fenugreek seeds for an Indian curry, or any of the other wide array of
ethnic dishes that come to us from around the world. Try to buy
U.S. grown herbs whenever possible, however, as most can easily
be grown locally.

Ethnic condiments bottled or canned elsewhere in the world
and imported into the United States exert a higher cost on the environment than imported spices. Because the contents are packaged
in liquid, the jars and containers are heavy to transport and take a
lot of space in transit. Instead of buying imported sauces and
condiments, search through ethnic cookbooks for recipes and
make your own.

HERBS

Herbs are plants whose leaves are rich in flavorful and aromatic essential oils. Herbs are used fresh and dried. Whenever possible use fresh herbs, as they have the most vibrant flavor, but in the winter, dried herbs can be used effectively, and they are a mainstay of a good pantry. (Parsley, cilantro, and basil lose their flavor when dried, but they can be frozen in season for the winter.) Generally, dried herbs have a stronger, more concentrated flavor.

Commonly used culinary herbs include sweet basil, bay leaves, chervil, chives, cilantro, dill, fennel, lemon balm, lemongrass, marjoram, mint, oregano, parsley, rosemary, sage, savory, tarragon, and thyme.

TIPS FOR USING HERBS

- ❋ To substitute fresh for dried herbs in a recipe, add three or four times more fresh herbs than the recipe calls for, and usually add at the end of the recipe.
- ❋ Experiment with soaking dried herbs for ten minutes or so before adding to a dish. Soak in water that has just boiled or the hot liquid used for cooking. (Heat releases the flavor of the herb.)
- ❋ Other than soaking herbs, before adding them to a recipe rub them between your fingers to release the essential oils.

SPICES

Whereas herbs are derived from leaves, spices are dried seeds, pods, roots, and other plant parts that are usually ground to fine powders. Spices include allspice, anise pepper (Szechuan pepper), caraway seeds, cardamom seeds, cassia, celery seed, cinnamon, clove, coriander, cumin, dill seed, fennel seed, fenugreek seed, ginger, lemongrass, mace, mustard seed, nutmeg, pepper, saffron, star anise, and turmeric.

TIPS FOR BUYING AND STORING HERBS AND SPICES

Whenever possible, buy the whole herb leaf or the whole spice plant part. Once either the leaf or plant part is broken or ground, a lot of flavor is lost. Instead, grind spices at home with a mortar and pestle, right before use. Dried herbs also can be crumbled in your hand, or easily broken apart, before using.

The best time to buy herbs and spices is in the late fall, shortly after they have been harvested. Store them in a cool, dry, dark cupboard, in airtight containers. Freezers also work well for storing herbs and spices.

HERB AND SPICE BLENDS

One secret of distinguishing oneself as a good cook is knowing how to use herbs and spices properly. When used well, herbs and spices can dazzle the taste buds, enhancing all the flavors in the food. If you like the idea of cooking from scratch with the basics—using foods from the pantry and fresh vegetables in season—or if you already do so, the big challenge is to master the art of flavoring.

Starting a notebook of herb blends for cuisines that appeal to you will reap real rewards. Every time you see a recipe in a magazine or cookbook that has a spice combination you like, write it down!

COMMONLY USED HERB AND SPICE COMBINATIONS

Bouquet Garni for Soups: Thyme, parsley, bay leaf, dill, tarragon.

Chinese Five-Spice Powder: Szechuan peppercorns, cinnamon, cloves, fennel, star anise, cassia.

Cajun Spices: Paprika, chili, garlic, allspice, thyme, cayenne.

Chili Powder: garlic, oregano, allspice, cloves, cumin seed, coriander seed, cayenne, black pepper, turmeric, mustard seed, paprika.

Creole Seasoning: Paprika, garlic, thyme, cayenne, oregano.

Desserts: Cinnamon, cloves, coriander, ginger, nutmeg, mace, cardamom.

French: Chives, chervil, parsley, thyme, tarragon.

Garam Masala / Indian Dishes: Cumin, coriander, cardamom, black pepper.

Indian Curry: Coriander seeds, cumin, nutmeg, cardamom seed, turmeric, white mustard seed, black mustard seed, fenugreek seed, chilis, ginger, peppercorns, garlic, allspice, cinnamon, cayenne, fennel.

Italian Blends: Oregano, basil, marjoram, tarragon, parsley,

Japanese Seven Flavors (Two Hot, Five Aromatic): Anise pepper, sesame seeds, flaxseeds, rapeseeds, poppy seeds, dried tangerine or orange peel, ground nori seaweed.

Mexican Combinations: Garlic, cumin, black pepper, cloves, oregano, cilantro, sometimes cinnamon and coriander.

Mexican Fajita: Ginger, paprika, jalapeño pepper, oregano, mustard, cumin, red pepper, parsley.

North and East African Flavors: Paprika, cumin, cloves, cardamom, peppercorns, allspice, fenugreek seeds, coriander seeds, ginger, turmeric, cinnamon, cloves.

Panch Phoron/Five Mixed Spices: Cumin, fennel, bay leaf, fenugreek, onion seeds.

Note: Coriander, cumin, and ginger, when used in combination with beans, reportedly diminish flatulence.

GUIDE TO HERBS AND SPICES

ALLSPICE

A member of the pepper family, it is so named because it naturally combines the flavors of a lot of other spices such as clove, cinnamon, and nutmeg.

Uses: Desserts, quick breads, pickling

ANISE

Tastes slightly like licorice.

> Uses: Added to salad, eggs, cheese, stews, and pastries; combines well with cinnamon and bay leaves

ANISE PEPPER (SZECHUAN PEPPER)

Not actually a pepper, but very hot.

> Uses: Chinese five-spice powder

BASIL

Green leaf that is highly fragrant and flavorful.

> Uses: Tomato dishes of all sorts, pesto (fresh leaves ideal), Italian, Mediterranean dishes; combines well with garlic, thyme, parsley, and oregano

BAY LEAF

Long thin leaf about two inches long; brittle when dried.

> Uses: Soups, sauces, stews, beans, marinades; combines well with basil, oregano, thyme, garlic, and pepper

CARAWAY SEEDS

Small, strong, and nutty-tasting seed.

> Uses: Commonly added to breads, vegetables, eggs, and cheeses

CARDAMOM SEEDS

Fragrant; sweet and slightly gingery flavor.

> Uses: Soups, stews, sweet potatoes, yams, white and red potatoes, and pastries; combines well with cumin and coriander
>
> *Tip:* For freshest flavor, buy cardamom seed pods, not ground

cardamom, then open to the small inner black seeds and grind yourself or use whole.

CASSIA

Often called Chinese cinnamon.
    Uses: Chinese five-spice powder

CELERY SEED

A very strong celery flavor.
    Uses: Vegetables, soups, sauces

CHERVIL

Subtle flavor well suited for less flavorful foods.
    Uses: Soups, stews, fish, and dairy products; combines well
        with parsley, tarragon, leeks, potatoes, and onions

CHIVES

Strong flavor of onions, but less hot.
    Uses: Potato, leek, or onion dishes; garnishes for vegetables and
        soups, bean dishes, salads; combines well with garlic,
        dill, marjoram, tarragon, and dairy products

CINNAMON

Fragrant with a rich, strong taste.
    Uses: Squashes, apples and other fruit, spice blends native to
        Asia and the Mediterranean; combines well with nutmeg,
        ginger, cloves, and cardamom

CLOVES

Very pungent and fragrant.
    Uses: Squashes, fruit, spice blends native to Asia and the

Mediterranean; combines well with cinnamon, nutmeg, and ginger

CORIANDER (ALSO KNOWN AS CILANTRO)

Seeds, leaves, root. Pungent flavor.
> Uses: Salsas, beans (Mexican dishes), Indian cuisine, salads, vegetables

CUMIN

Seed with a very strong, rich flavor.
> Uses: Beans, vegetables, curries

DILL

Very strong herbal flavor.
> Uses: Soups, salads, vegetables such as tomatoes and cucumbers, dairy products, crepes, bland-tasting foods such as cauliflower, potatoes; dill stands alone and does not need other herbs

FENNEL SEEDS

Sometimes confused with anise, as the licorice flavor is similar but milder.
> Uses: Salads, tomatoes, grains, beans, dairy products

FENUGREEK

Most frequently used in combination with other spices.
> Uses: Curries, African dishes

GARLIC

Pungent, onionlike flavor.
> Uses: Salad dressings, ethnic dishes of all sorts (Italian in particular)

GINGER

Pungent and flavorful root.
>   Uses: Baked goods, desserts, ethnic cuisine from Asia and Africa

LEMON BALM

Fragrant leaf that tastes like lemon.
>   Uses: Vegetables, beans, desserts; any recipes where lemon can be used
>   *Note:* Fresh is far preferable for flavor.

LEMONGRASS

A strong citrus aroma and flavor; the stems and roots are used.
>   Uses: Broths, marinades, infused oils, salads; combines well with ginger, chili, and coconut

MACE

The "jacket" of the nutmeg. The flavor is milder than nutmeg.
>   Uses: Desserts, sauces

MARJORAM

A strongly flavored small leaf.
>   Uses: Italian and other Mediterranean dishes, but it can be added to most vegetables, salad dressings, stews, and sauces; combines well with oregano, basil, and tarragon

MINT

Mint is very refreshing, which is why it is used so frequently in drinks on hot days.
>   Uses: Tea, jelly, beans, grain or potato salads

MUSTARD

There are a number of different varieties of mustard: white, yellow, brown, and black. Mild (white) to hot (black), mustard has a tangy and spicy flavor.

Uses: Vinaigrette salad dressings, "mustard," Indian dishes

NUTMEG

Rich nutty flavor.

Uses: Desserts such as pumpkin pie, puddings, cakes, cookies

OREGANO

A hearty-flavored herb, popular from Italian cuisine.

Uses: Tomato sauces, cheese, minestrone-type soups, vegetables; combines well with garlic, parsley, thyme, basil, tarragon, and marjoram

PARSLEY

A spicy-tasting green leaf.

Uses: Garnish, grain and potato dishes, pastas, pesto, salads

PEPPER

Cayenne

Poignant and fiery hot.

Uses: Sauces, soups, beans, chiles; Mexican, Cajun, and Creole dishes; combines well with chilis

Note: Cayenne becomes more flavorful when it is frozen. Cayenne is very high in vitamin C and vitamin A.

Chili

Very hot and spicy.

Uses: Beans, eggs; chili powder may be a blend of chili, oregano, cumin, and other herbs and spices

Paprika

Flavorful pepper that is not as hot as cayenne or chilis.
Uses: European, African, Portuguese, and Spanish recipes

Peppercorns

There are black and white peppercorns; the white are ripened.

ROSEMARY

A thin twiglike leaf with a strong flavor often associated with poultry stuffing, and roast pork and potatoes.
Uses: Bread stuffing, vegetables, salad dressings, sauces, soups; combines well with thyme, parsley, and bay leaf

SAFFRON

Red "threads" with a fragrant flavor. The stamen of a purple flowering crocus, saffron is the most expensive spice in the world.
Uses: Rice, Indian and North African cuisines

SAGE

Small gray-green leaves; strong, hearty flavor.
Uses: Mostly used on meats but also on potatoes and in stuffings and breads

SAVORY

Aromatic herb similar to thyme and rosemary.
Uses: Beans, vegetables, teas, vinegars

STAR ANISE

A seed pod that is shaped like a star, it has a strong taste of licorice.
Uses: Chinese five-spice powder

TARRAGON

Strong and distinctive herb, a little goes a long way.
Uses: Mushrooms, leeks, potatoes, peas, dairy products, salad
dressings

THYME

Small gray-green leaves with a spicy, pinelike flavor.
Uses: Beans, soups, stews, vegetables, garnish, dairy products

TURMERIC

Vivid yellow spice with a spicy flavor.
Uses: Indian dishes, curries

VANILLA

Bean is split open and placed with a liquid such as alcohol for
steeping.
Uses: Desserts of all kinds

TEAS

A prized herbalist in her community in upstate New York, Fara
Shaw Kelsey is enlightening about which herbal teas to have in
one's home and why. Confused by the wide array of herbal tea mix-
tures available in stores, and not knowing what to choose, we asked
her for advice on how to make sense of them all. She generously
invited me over to "share the ritual of drinking tea, something that
is a ritual in all cultures" and to talk about teas.

Ensconced in her cozy kitchen, with a root vegetable stew simmering gently on the stove (it was winter), drinking a blueberry leaf
tea, she began to weave the story of how healthful and healing
herbal teas are. Extolling the virtues of nettle, dandelion root, and
fennel teas, she opened up a world unknown to me. Most of us
think of dandelions and nettles primarily as only being weeds. Fara

is urging us to look at these plants in a way different from the way we had before, as healing foods.

Herbalists use the term *simples* to describe herbs utilized one species at a time instead of as complex formulas. After Fara described simples, they seemed to me an excellent starting point for a beginner herbal tea maker, and it is an approach she recommends. In fact, she advises that people not get involved—either in buying or making one's own—in complex tea formulas unless they are very sophisticated about what the herbs are being used for. I heard this with relief as I thought of the basket of herbal tea blends that are on top of the refrigerator in my home. Overwhelmed by my lack of knowledge, I had found these teas intimidating. For all I knew, my family could be drinking stimulating drinks before sleep, and sleepy drinks for breakfast!

Fara has nine simples she recommends for every pantry. They are mint, fennel, dandelion leaf and root, echinacea, nettle, blueberry leaf, ginger root, and the caffeinated green and flowering jasmine teas. Other herbs she likes are oatstraw, red clover, and cardamom. She suggests we buy the herbal teas in bulk in health food stores or from special mail-order suppliers (see "Resources"), and make sure they are either organic or wild crafted (that is, harvested in the wild). Bulk herbs are found either packaged or in jars for you to serve yourself how much you need. If unpackaged, make sure the herb has retained some of its aroma or it may be too old. Fara suggests making the herbs into infusions, as described below, but if you are really busy she says most health food stores now sell the herbs in tea bag form. All dried herbs should be stored in a dry, dark glass or a dark cupboard or closet.

A lovely part of my visit with Fara was sharing a pot of tea and experiencing the relaxing benefits of the tea ritual. "Come and have a cup of tea with me" is an invitation we could all benefit from in our busy lives. And if the tea you offer is a unique homemade herbal infusion, so much the better. If we start looking at herbs as potential teas, we begin looking at the environment just out our front doors in a different way, becoming more aware of the plants around us and newly perceiving weeds as nutrient-rich foods for our families.

How to Make Herbal Tea Infusions

Take a handful of the dried herb and put it in a glass jar (such as a mason jar or wide-mouthed glass coffeepot). Pour boiling water over that (put a stainless steel knife into the jar to absorb some of the heat so that the jar doesn't crack) and immediately stir the herb, making sure all the plant material is wet. Quickly cover the jar so that the vapors do not escape. (The vapors are full of the plant's volatile oils, which you want to keep in your tea.) Let the jar sit at room temperature for four hours, or until completely cooled. Place in the refrigerator. Fara makes her infusions right before going to bed at night and leaves them out on the counter to cool until morning. Before drinking, strain the tea and serve hot or at room temperature.

Guide to Herbal Teas

BLUEBERRY LEAF

Used by the American Indians, blueberry leaf is reportedly the herb of choice for helping to control blood sugar problems and varicose veins. Because it has a delicious flavor, the tea has culinary as well as medicinal uses.

DANDELION ROOT

Fara thinks everyone can benefit from dandelion root, leaves, and even flowers. Highly nutritious, dandelion root is known as a tonic, which means it can help heal disease. Reportedly a strong diuretic, it is also high in the minerals iron, manganese, phosphorous, magnesium, calcium, chromium, cobalt, zinc, and potassium. Considered one of the all-time best herbs for the liver, it is said to help the body remove poisons.

ECHINACEA ROOT

The reported healing properties of echinacea root were discovered by the American Indians, who used it to help heal wounds.

Herbalists regard echinacea as a great boon to the immune system, helping to fight off viral and even some bacterial infections.

FENNEL

Originating in the Mediterranean, fennel is widely grown in the United States. It has a taste like licorice, and for that reason Fara chooses it for children. It is a pleasant tea to have for dinner, and an excellent natural breath freshener. Both seeds and leaves are used for teas. They are both considered excellent for the intestinal tract.

FLOWERING JASMINE TEA

Fara recommends this tea because of the beauty of the flowers floating in it. Originating in China, it also grows in the southern United States. Flowering jasmine tea includes the jasmine flowers along with the tea leaves. When water is added they are revitalized and float in the tea. An elegant enhancement for special occasions. (See "Resources" for sources.)

GINGER ROOT

Slice off a piece of root, pour boiling water over it, let steep for ten or fifteen minutes, and drink with a little honey or other whole food sweetener. Ginger is reportedly very helpful for digestion. It helps digest fats, helps the circulation, and has a very warming effect, so it is a great winter tea.

GREEN TEA

The tea used in traditional Japanese tea ceremonies, green tea has been extolled by Buddhist monks for being a miraculous medicine for maintaining health and for having extraordinary powers to promote longevity. Green tea's tannin contains catechin, and studies reveal that catechin and green tea reportedly help reduce cancers of the esophagus and stomach, reduce high blood sugar, high blood pressure, decrease the buildup of serum cholesterol (LDL) while having a minimal effect on HDL cholesterol. If these attributes weren't inspiring enough, green tea also is a breath freshener and contains natural fluorine, which helps to fight cavities.

MINT

A very refreshing tea, it is also a bit stimulating. Considered a soothing nerve tonic, it reportedly can also help stimulate digestion. Mint tea is delightful whether served cold on hot summer days or hot in the winter.

NETTLE

Fara couldn't rave enough about nettle. An incredibly nutritious plant, stinging nettle is high in chromium, cobalt, iron, phosphorous, zinc, copper, and sulfur, as well as B complex vitamins, especially thiamin and riboflavin. Herbalists believe nettle helps restore adrenal and kidney function, stabilize blood sugar, and restore overall health. It is reportedly also a great preventive for those who want to maintain good health. Last but not least, nettle is an excellent composter, and it is used in biodynamic compost for this reason. Once cooked, stinging nettle loses its bite.

WHOLE FOOD SWEETENERS

Making the switch from white sugar to whole food sweeteners can be a difficult one, especially if you have to please children who have become used to desserts sweetened with white sugar. But desserts made with whole food sweeteners can be delicious. The flavors are more delicate than desserts made with sugar.

GUIDE TO MILDLY REFINED SWEETENERS

BARLEY AND OTHER GRAIN MALTS

Derived from a natural process that sprouts, heats, and dries barley. Considered the most preferable sweetener by many macrobiotics, grain malts are close to being a whole food and are not overly sweet or highly concentrated.

DATE SUGAR

Made from dehydrated ground dates. Does not dissolve well in liquids.

FRUIT JUICE CONCENTRATES

Made from the juice of apples, grapes, pears, and/or oranges, which has been reduced by about one-quarter by slow cooking. By freezing fruit juice concentrates, and drying fruits during times of their harvest, you can keep your family supplied with sugar substitutes until next year's harvest.

GRANULAR FRUIT SWEETENERS

White grape juice and grain sweeteners that have been dehydrated and granulated.

HONEY

A whole food made by bees from flower nectar. Although it is not refined by humans, it is actually highly refined by the bees. It has very few nutrients but more nutrients than refined sugar. Honey has also been found to have medicinal value when added to tea when treating colds and cold symptoms. Be aware, however, that honey and corn syrup should never be given to infants, whose digestive tracts are prone to the growth of a deadly toxin produced by the botulism spores found in these substances.

MALTOSE

Sprouted grains and cooked rice, heated and fermented until starch turns to sugar. Available in Chinese markets.

MAPLE SYRUP

Boiled-down sap of maple trees. It takes forty gallons of sap to make one gallon of syrup. Though this process evaporates the water from the sap, it retains the minerals, and, ounce for ounce, maple syrup has twice as much calcium as milk!

MOLASSES

Unsulfured molasses is made from the juice of sun-ripened cane; sulfured molasses is a by-product of refined sugar; blackstrap molasses is the residue of the cane syrup after the sugar crystals have been separated. It is very nutritious, with high levels of calcium, iron, and potassium.

RICE SYRUP

Made from rice and sprouted grains.

SORGHUM SYRUP

Sorghum cane juice, boiled to a syrup. Sorghum cane tends to need few pesticides because it is naturally resistant to insects.

STEVIA

A plant native to the Americas, with sweet leaves and buds. According to Paul Pitchford, author of *Healing with Whole Foods*, stevia has thirty times the sweetness of sugar with almost no calories. Pitchford recommends one to three drops of stevia to sweeten one cup of liquid. Stevia is increasingly available in health food stores and is found as either a powder or liquid extract.

SUCANAT

Sucanat is a product developed by Dr. Max-Henri Beguin, a pediatrician from Switzerland. The makers of Sucanat report that though

Natural Sweetener Equivalents to ½ Cup White or Brown Sugar

Equivalent	½ Cup Sugar
White/brown sugar	½ cup
Barley malt	1½ cups
Date sugar	1 cup
Fruit juice	½ cup
Concentrate	
Granular Fruit	½ cup
Sweeteners	
Honey	⅓ cup
Maltose	1¼ cups
Maple syrup	½ cup
Molasses	⅓ cup
Rice syrup	1¼ cups
Sorghum syrup	⅓ cup
Sucanat	½ cup

Sucanat, like sugar, is made from sugarcane juice, nothing is added to or taken out of the juice except water. Sucanat thus reportedly retains all of the minerals, vitamins, and trace elements from the sugarcane, containing, for instance, 1125 milligrams of potassium (sugar contains 4.5 milligrams) and 1600 I.U. of vitamin A. The retained nutrients make Sucanat a much better choice than sugar.

TIPS

When you substitute liquid sweeteners for dry, reduce or eliminate the liquid content of the recipe, and increase the flour to taste. For breads and pies, flavorful fruit juice concentrates and other liquid sweeteners such as maple syrup work very well.

When a recipe doesn't call for any liquid, choose a dry, granular sweetener like date sugar or Sucanat, or what you're baking will be too breadlike from the additional flour needed for proper consistency. For cakes and cupcakes that need to resemble "the real thing," choose sorghum syrup or Sucanat.

Sweets made with whole food sweeteners tend to have a slightly more subtle sweetness than sweets made with white or brown sugar. If you miss the clearly defined sweetness that comes from a more refined sugar, try adding a tart fruit, such as cranberries, where appropriate (with muffins, for instance), or a bit more spice like cinnamon in a coffee cake or cookie recipe. Sometimes the best sweet isn't a cookie but a piece of fruit, which doesn't taste like its artificial counterpart.

HEALTHFUL OILS

Oils are pressed from the seeds and fruit of plants. Unrefined oils are the most nutritious, as they have not been stripped of fat-soluble vitamins A, D, E, and K. They are also the most flavorful, tasting of the nut or seed they have been pressed from. Refined oils, especially those that are mass-marketed, are nutritionally depleted, and the essential fatty acids are damaged from the high-heat processing; they are extracted with solvents, refined with chemicals, and contain preservatives. Refined oils have very little flavor.

Superunsaturated and polyunsaturated unrefined oils such as canola, soy, walnut, and flax oils contain omega-3 and omega-6 essential fatty acids, which are essential to good health. (See chapter 2 for a more detailed explanation.) Unrefined oils highest in omega-3 and omega-6, in descending order, are hemp, flax, pumpkin, canola, walnut, soybean, safflower, sunflower, sesame, rice bran, and almond. Unrefined monounsaturated oils, such as canola, olive, and high-oleic safflower oils, are also important for health and are linked to reducing serum cholesterol. Saturated oils are considered unhealthful oils and are primarily made up of animal fat, although nuts contain some saturated fats. All plant oils are cholesterol free.

Unfortunately, unrefined oils are very fragile and change at a molecular level when heated, making them smoke and release toxic fumes. Refined oils, on the other hand, especially those high in monounsaturates, can withstand high heat before breaking down and smoking. It is important to have three kinds of oil in your kitchen: unrefined oils rich in omega-3 and omega-6 to be used in salad dressings and in sauces that are simmered, steeped, and stewed; unrefined olive oil high in monounsaturated fats for medium-heat cooking; and a refined oil high in monounsaturates, such as high-oleic safflower oil, for high-heat cooking.

Unrefined, polyunsaturated, and superunsaturated oils begin to smoke above 375°F. They also have a higher moisture content and fizz at higher temperatures, and important nutrients such as vitamin E are destroyed. Unrefined oils higher in monounsaturated fats such as olive, sesame, corn, peanut, and safflower oils can be heated from 255°F to 350°F. Only refined oils should be used for temperatures above 350°F. Refined canola, peanut, safflower, sunflower, and walnut oils can be used between 325°F and 400°F. Refined high-oleic safflower and avocado oils are ideal for high-heat cooking of temperatures up to 520°F. (See table on page 173.)

In terms of cost to the environment, oils are very expensive. It takes almost two thousand olives to make just a quart of olive oil, for example, and a great deal of land to support the trees that produce the olives. Eating nuts and seeds themselves can be the best way of getting your essential fatty acids, and is less burdensome for the environment. When you do use oils, try to use them sparingly, and as much as you can, try to eliminate high-heat cooking that requires refined oils.

CHOICES IN HOW THE FRUITS AND SEEDS ARE PRESSED

Different methods are used to extract the oil out of fruits and seeds. Some methods are purer than others; the best choice is an oil that is 100 percent expeller or mechanically pressed. Once the oil is removed, however, it can then be further refined. Only the label will tell you if the oil is refined or not.

Expeller-Pressed/Mechanically Pressed: Oil that has been extracted from the seed mechanically, as opposed to chemically. Expeller-pressed oils are usually found in health food stores. Also, the heat used to expel the oil remains below 200°F, thereby not reducing the healthful fat-soluble nutrients such as vitamin E.

Cold-Pressed: See Expeller-Pressed. Oils that are pressed at temperatures that do not rise above 120°F.

Solvent-Extracted: A chemical method of extracting oil from fruits and seeds. Hexane is the most common chemical used in solvent extraction. Some hexane can be found in solvent-extracted oils. Oils that have been extracted by solvents are considered refined oils.

Refined: Oil that has been extracted by solvents. Refined oils are often stripped of oil's naturally occurring vitamin E, which can act as a natural preventative against rancidity.

STORAGE OF OILS

Light causes free radicals to develop in oils, oxygen causes rancidity, and heat affects the molecular structure. Store oil in a cool location until the bottle is opened, and once opened, place it in the refrigerator. Unrefined oils go rancid more quickly than refined. Once refrigerated, unrefined oils can last between five and ten months, and refined oils up to twenty months. If you go through some oils very slowly consider freezing them. In the freezer unrefined oils can last up to twelve months. Rancid oils smell stale and can taste bitter.

GUIDE TO OILS

ALMOND OIL

Most commonly available refined.

Cooking Methods and Their Temperatures

Below 212°F: Boil, steam, scald, stew, simmer, steep, parboil, salad dressings.

Below 320°F: Low-heat baking, light sauté, pressure cooking.

Below 375°F: Baking, sauté, stir-fry, wok cooking.

Below 500°F: Sear, brown, deep-fry, fry.

Fatty Acid Profile: Nine percent saturated, 65 percent monounsaturated, 26 percent polyunsaturated
Smoke Point/Refined Oil: 495°F

AVOCADO OIL

Refined, it can be heated to the highest temperature of all the plant oils.

Fatty Acid Profile: Twenty percent saturated, 70 percent
monounsaturated, 10 percent polyunsaturated
Smoke Point/Refined Oil: 520°F

CANOLA OIL

Canola has the lowest amount of saturated fat of any of the oils and also contains both omega-6 and omega-3 oils.

Unrefined

Fatty Acid Profile: Six percent saturated, 60 percent monounsaturated, 24 percent polyunsaturated, 10 percent superunsaturated (contains omega-3)
Smoke Point: Below 225°F

Semirefined

Smoke Point: 350°F

Refined

Smoke Point: 400°F

CORN OIL

Corn and safflower oils are the only oils indigenous to North America.

Unrefined

> Fatty Acid Profile: Thirteen percent saturated, 27 percent monounsaturated, 60 percent polyunsaturated
> Smoke Point: Below 320°F

Refined

> Smoke Point: 450°F

FLAXSEED OIL

Contains 57 percent superunsaturated omega-3 essential fatty acids, the highest of any oils. Frequently used medicinally for this reason.

Unrefined

> Fatty Acid Profile: Nine percent saturated, 16 percent monounsaturated, 18 percent polyunsaturated, 57 percent superunsaturated
> Smoke Point: Below 225°F

OLIVE OIL

Contains 82 percent of monounsaturated fatty acids, the highest of any of the oils. Monounsaturates are heralded as helpers in the fight against heart disease.

Unrefined

> Fatty Acid Profile: Ten percent saturated, 82 percent monounsaturated, 8 percent polyunsaturated
> Smoke Point: Below 320°F

Note: The best olive oil is produced from the fruit of the olive trees grown in the Mediterranean region. Because olive oil comes from the soft pulp of the fruit rather than from a seed it needs no high-pressure extraction and can thus truly be considered "cold-pressed."

Olives are crushed in a mill that breaks the pulp but not the pits. The first extraction is a gentle pressing that does not heat the oil much beyond room temperature. The oil is then separated from the olive pulp. Oil obtained from this first pressing is the only oil that can be called "virgin" olive oil.

"Virgin" olive oil comes in three grades: "extra-virgin," "fine virgin," and plain "virgin." The difference is solely one of taste and acidity, with the plain "virgin" having the highest acid content and the "extra-virgin" having the lowest.

"Pure" olive oil is still 100 percent olive oil but it is not "virgin." In other words, "pure olive oil" is extracted from second pressings, which require higher temperatures for extraction or solvent extraction. For this reason it is not the best choice.

PEANUT OIL

Unrefined peanut oil is very flavorful for a light sauté.

Unrefined

> Fatty Acid Profile: Nineteen percent saturated, 51 percent monounsaturated, 30 percent polyunsaturated
> Smoke Point: Below 320°F

Refined

> Smoke Point: 450°F

SAFFLOWER OIL

Of all oils, safflower oil is the highest in polyunsaturated fatty acids.

Unrefined

> Fatty Acid Profile: Eight percent saturated, 13 percent monounsaturated, 79 percent polyunsaturated
> Smoke Point: 225°F

Semirefined

Smoke Point: Below 320°F

Refined

Smoke Point: Below 450°F

HIGH-OLEIC SAFFLOWER OIL

The fatty acid profile of this oil is completely different from that of regular safflower oil.

Unrefined

Fatty Acid Profile: Eight percent saturated, 76 percent monounsaturated, 16 percent polyunsaturated
Smoke Point: Below 320°F

Refined

Smoke Point: 450°F

SESAME OIL

Unrefined oil is an excellent choice for flavorful light sautés.

Unrefined

Fatty Acid Profile: Thirteen percent saturated, 46 percent monounsaturated, 41 percent polyunsaturated
Smoke Point: Below 350°F

Semirefined

Smoke Point: Below 450°F

SOY OIL

A good source of omega-3 essential fatty acids.

Unrefined

Fatty Acid Profile: Fourteen percent saturated, 28 percent monounsaturated, 50 percent polyunsaturated, 8 percent superunsaturated omega-3

Smoke Point: Below 320°F

Semirefined

Smoke Point: Below 350°F

Refined

Smoke Point: 450°F

SUNFLOWER OIL

Unrefined

Fatty Acid Profile: Twelve percent saturated, 19 percent monounsaturated, 69 percent polyunsaturated

Smoke Point: 225°F

Semirefined

Smoke Point: 450°F

HIGH-OLEIC SUNFLOWER OIL

Very similar to the fatty acid profile of olive oil.

Unrefined

Fatty Acid Profile: Eight percent saturated, 81 percent monounsaturated, 11 percent polyunsaturated

Smoke Point: Below 320°F

Refined

Smoke Point: 450°F

WALNUT OIL

Excellent for salad dressings, as it is a good source of omega-3 essential fatty acids.

Unrefined

Fatty Acid Profile: Sixteen percent saturated, 28 percent monounsaturated, 49 percent polyunsaturated, 5 percent superunsaturated omega-3

Smoke Point: Under 320°F

Semirefined

Smoke Point: 400°F

Preserving the Foods
of the Harvest

While it isn't difficult to buy local, even organic produce during harvest time, it is hard and expensive to maintain a diet of those foods in the winter and early spring. Yet after savoring the flavors of fresh foods and enjoying their environmental and health benefits, it can be frustrating to switch back to lackluster supermarket produce. One viable way of solving this problem is to preserve local food in season. Food preservation is perhaps the most useful tool for establishing a green kitchen year-round, and the rewards are immense. Opening a jar of dried tomatoes in the middle of a January snowstorm to add to a pasta, or spreading strawberry jam you made yourself on toast for your children, is very satisfying. It is a treat in the winter to know where your food came from.

For the most part, the days of preserving food by standing over a hot stove canning for two weeks straight during the dog days of August are long gone. Most people nowadays approach preserving food in an eclectic way, according to taste and time. A popular combination of techniques people tend to use is freezing most fruits, vegetables, and ready-made foods like tomato sauces; drying tomatoes and vegetables for winter soups, and fruit for children's snacks; pickling cucumbers; preserving berries; canning tomatoes (it takes one full day to can fifty quarts of tomatoes); and, if there is space, using cold storage for root vegetables. The popularity of this combination of preserving techniques is not surprising: it is manageable for even very busy lives, and it keeps food preservation interesting.

This chapter is designed to help you understand the concept behind different sorts of food-preserving procedures, and gauge the cost of equipment and the amount of time needed, so that you can mix and match techniques according to your personal tastes and circumstances. If you live in the city, the only thing that will be hard for you to manage is making a root cellar, though I'm told it has been done! No matter what techniques you choose, if you preserve food when it is bountiful and cheap, you will save a lot of money on your grocery bill in the winter (recovering the cost of the equipment quickly) and eliminate many trips to the store, which will save gas and time. Start with a manageable project, and every year you can add more skills to your repertoire.

THE SECRETS OF FOOD PRESERVATION

There are two processes that cause food to decay: enzyme activity and the growth of microorganisms. In order for these two processes to flourish, they need a suitable environment of air, moisture, heat, and acid content. Food preservation halts or retards enzyme activity and the growth of microorganisms by manipulating the food's exposure to these elements, which feed the decay process.

STOPPING THE GROWTH OF MICROORGANISMS

When produce is picked, microorganisms (bacteria, yeasts, and molds) slowly but surely start growing on it, ultimately making the food inedible and sometimes even poisonous. But microorganisms are all affected by heat, oxygen, moisture, and acid content. Each preserving technique manipulates these elements, and thereby the microorganisms, in a different way. Canning, for example, heats the food to such a high temperature that the microorganisms are killed. (The reason that high heat processing is so important for canning is that some bacteria, like *C. botulinum,* thrive in an oxygen-free environment, as is found in a jar of canned vegetables. The jar needs to be heated to a temperature high enough to kill *C. botulinum.*) Freezing, on the other hand, reduces the temperature to such a degree that the multiplication of microorganisms is halted. Drying sucks the moisture out of the food so that microorganisms can't grow, but it isn't as successful at halting microorganisms as the freezing technique, as anyone with mold allergies can testify. Since microorganisms do not thrive in acidic environments, pickling is another successful preservation technique.

STOPPING THE ENZYME PROCESS

Enzymes cause chemical transformations that ripen fruits and vegetables and also cause them to decay after being picked. The chemical process of decay needs to be halted in order to preserve the food for the future. Only heat, freezing, or a highly acidic environment can halt enzyme activity. Moisture and oxygen halt the growth of microorganisms but have no effect on enzymes.

Time is an important factor to consider in working to halt the enzyme process after ripening. The sooner after picking that a food is processed for preserving, the better. Food that is cut open has to be tended to immediately if you want to preserve it. The sooner it is plunged into a blanching hot water or steam bath, for example, or the sooner fruit is treated with ascorbic acid or citric acid, the less enzyme damage your food will have. After treatment, one needs to freeze, dry, or can the food quickly. Enzymes work at different speeds for different fruits and vegetables. A cool root cellar halts enzymes just enough to keep a potato for a number of months, but a strawberry would hardly last a few days and needs to be frozen or canned. (See the table "Preservation Techniques" page 184, for a list of which techniques are appropriate for which foods.)

GENERAL GUIDELINES FOR PRESERVING FOOD

The three rules of thumb for preserving food are to be scrupulously clean, to follow directions to the letter, and to work fast (except for preparing food for root cellars). Contaminated food is no joke. Nor is food that has lost all its nutritive value because of improper handling. While canning is the procedure with the most danger of deadly food poisoning if done improperly, all techniques must be approached responsibly. This being said, you should not be frightened away from

The Demise of Microorganisms and Enzymes

	Microorganisms	Enzymes
Heat		
	Halted below 32°F	Cold slows—but does not halt—process
	Retarded 32–50°F	Cold slows process
	Thrive 50–120°F	Thrive 85–120°F
	Stopped 212–240°F* in high-acid foods	Thrive 85–120°F
	Killed 240°F in low-acid foods	Inactivated 240°F
Moisture		
	Halted when below 35 percent	No effect
	Thrive when damp	
	Retarded when saturated	
Acidity		
	Hostile environment	Slows process
Sugar		
	Hostile environment	
Salt		
	Hostile environment	
Oxygen		
	Most thrive in air	No effect
	C. botulinum grows with no oxygen	

It is essential that canned foods be heated to 240°F for the appropriate amount of time (see page 181) to kill the deadly C. botulinum.

"putting food by," as experienced preservers like to say. Fortunately, if the three rules of thumb of food preservation are followed, you should be guaranteed excellent, flavorful, and healthful results.

Preservation Techniques

Technique	How It Works
Freezing	Cold stops enzyme process and growth of microorganisms; food is stored in airtight containers.
Drying	Removes moisture; food heated.
Root Cellars	Slows enzyme process and the growth of microorganisms by reducing temperature to 32–35°F for most foods, 50–60°F for others.
Canning	
Boiling water bath	Oxygen is removed; the food is processed at a high heat; and the food must be acidic.
Pressure canner	Oxygen is removed; the food is processed at a very high heat (240°F).
Jams and Jellies	Oxygen is removed; the food is acidic and sweetened; it is processed at a high heat.
Pickling	Usually oxygen is removed; high-acid content; usually processed at a high heat.
Smoking*	Salt reduces growth of bacteria and pulls out moisture; sugar curing reduces growth of bacteria; smoke coats the meat, protecting it from rancidity; the food is dried.
Curing*	Salt and sugar both reduce growth of bacteria; salt pulls out moisture; the food is dried.

Due to the high salt content of curing and smoking and the health concerns of by-products of smoke, neither process is recommended as a healthful means of food preservation.

If you are at a high altitude (above five thousand feet), you must follow directions specific to your location for blanching and canning times. Call your county's cooperative extension service. These offices are funded in every state by the federal government, are administered by state agricultural colleges, and generally have a specialist in food preservation. Ask them for guidelines for home preserving at your altitude.

PRETREATMENTS

Most of the fruits and vegetables that are to be prepared for drying, freezing, and canning should be pretreated to halt the enzyme action and the early growth of microorganisms. Blanching heats water or steam to 212°F, the temperature needed to stop enzyme activity in acidic foods. Blanching is also recommended for most vegetables that are to be dried and canned. Fruit is typically pretreated using acids such as ascorbic acid (vitamin C) or citric acid to stop the enzyme process from browning the fruit once it has been cut.

BLANCHING

Blanching partially precooks vegetables by scalding them in boiling water or steam. It also halts the enzyme process. For these reasons blanching is highly recommended. Blanching will also help maintain the flavor of the vegetables.

There are two kinds of blanching: water blanching and steam blanching. With water blanching, food is plunged into, and covered by, rapidly boiling water. With steam blanching, the food is steamed at a high temperature. Steaming is the method that retains the most nutritive value in the food, but some foods, such as greens, mat together when steamed and need to be water blanched. Ironically, if food is not blanched for a long enough time, enzyme activity will be sped up. Overblanching, on the other hand, will result in the food losing some nutrient value as well as losing color, crispness, and flavor.

Water Blanching

Equipment

- ❋ A large pot with a tight-fitting cover, capable of holding two or more gallons of rapidly boiling water. The pot should be made of stainless steel or enamel.
- ❋ Cutting board, sharp knife, and a vegetable peeler.
- ❋ Wire basket/strainer insert to fit inside the pot; preferably two, one for ice bath (if freezing), one for boiling water bath. If you do not have a wire basket, cheesecloth will do,

but it does not allow as much water to circulate among the vegetables as a basket/strainer does.

Procedure

1. Clean cutting boards, knives, pot, and strainers.
2. Prepare and clean appropriate equipment (see under specific processing type: canning, freezing, or drying).
3. Fill the pot with water (about one gallon per pound of vegetables), add basket/strainer, and heat to a roiling boil.
4. Prepare produce by washing, trimming off stems, coring and slicing when appropriate, and cutting off bad spots.
5. Keeping the water at a full boil, quickly pull out the basket/strainer, fill with the vegetables (all one type), plunge into the boiling water, and quickly cover to maintain roiling boil.
6. Immediately set the timer for the appropriate number of minutes needed to blanch the particular vegetable you are processing. If the food is scalded for too long it will lose its crispness.
7. Once the time is up, pull the vegetables out of the boiling water and plunge them immediately into an ice water bath. (You will need a couple of trays of ice cubes per pound of vegetables.)
8. Once the vegetables are completely cold, process according to the directions under "Canning Food," "Food Freezing," or "Drying Food."

Steam Blanching

Equipment

* A large pot with a tight-fitting cover, capable of holding two or more gallons of rapidly boiling water. The pot should be made of stainless steel or enamel.
* Cutting board, sharp knife, and a vegetable peeler.
* A steamer tray (metal baskets available in kitchen stores) that fits into your large pot.
* It helps to have two wire baskets/strainers: one for the boiling water bath and one for the ice water bath.

Follow the procedure for water blanching, but instead of filling the pot with water, place the steamer on the bottom of the pot and fill with water to just cover the steamer, and once the steam is escaping, place one layer of vegetables at a time in the steamer.

Blanching Time for Vegetables

❋ For steam blanching, add one minute to the time recommended.

❋ Wait to start counting minutes until water is at a full boil again.

Vegetable	Blanching time (in minutes)
Artichokes, trimmed	4, small to medium (add juice of one lemon to blanching water)
Asparagus, ends	2–4, depending on size
Beans (lima)	3–4, depending on size
Beans (green)	3–4, depending on size
Beets, sliced	cook (in simmering water) until tender
Beet greens	2 (water blanch only)
Broccoli flowerets	2–4, depending on size
Brussels sprouts	3–5, depending on size
Cabbage wedges	3
Carrots	3–4, whole
Cauliflower flowerets	3–5, depending on size (add juice of one lemon to blanching water)
Celery, 1-inch lengths	3
Collard greens	3 (water blanch only)
Corn on the cob	5–7, depending on size
Corn, cut kernels	6–8
Cucumber slices	none, puree for freezing
Eggplant slices	4
Greens	3 (water blanch only)
Herbs	1
Kale	1 (water blanch only)
Kohlrabi	2 (small, whole), 1 (sliced)
Leek	none
Mushrooms, slices	2–4 (add juice of one lemon to blanching water)
Okra, unsliced	2–3, depending on size
Onions	none

Blanching Time for Vegetables (continued)

Vegetable	Blanching time (in minutes)
Parsley	15–20 seconds
Parsnips, sliced	2
Peas, shelled	1 minute, shelled
Peppers (green, red), halved	3 (optional)
Peppers (hot)	none
Potatoes	cook, baked, or fried
Pumpkin, cubed	cook
Rutabagas, sliced	2
Spinach	2 (water blanch only)
Squash, summer, sliced	3
Squash, winter	cook
Sweet potatoes	cook (dip in mild lemon juice solution before baking)
Swiss chard	2 (water blanch only)
Tomatoes	boil until skins crack; cool and remove skins; simmer (10 minutes)
Turnips, sliced	2

ACID TREATMENTS

If you add lemon juice to a freshly cut avocado or apple to keep them from browning, you are giving the fruit an acid treatment. Acid treatments reduce enzyme activity, creating a hostile environment for microorganisms. For these reasons, acid (vinegar or lemon juice) is used to pickle, for example. Acid treatments are used for freezing, drying, and canning many fruits and some vegetables.

For fruit, add acid to apples, avocados, bananas, cherries, mangoes, melons, nectarines, peaches, pears, and persimmons.

Equipment
* Stainless steel or enamel pans or bowls.
* Ascorbic acid, available in health food stores.
* Slotted spoon.

Procedure

The acid treatment of fruit varies, depending on whether you are canning, freezing, or drying. For canning, the extra acid is sometimes added to the packing liquid. The same is true for fruit frozen in a syrup. For drying fruit and freezing fruit without a syrup, however, observe the following procedure.

1. Clean cutting boards, knives, pot, strainers.
2. Prepare produce by washing, trimming off stems, coring and slicing when appropriate, and cutting off bad spots.
3. Place two quarts of cold water in pan or bowl (add three or four ice cubes).
4. Add three tablespoons lemon juice.
5. Add fruit (loosely packed, not crushed) to pan or bowl.
6. Leave in pan from one to five minutes.
7. Remove fruit with slotted spoon, and air dry.

FREEZING FOOD

Frozen food loses fewer vitamins and minerals in processing than any other of the preserved foods. The faster it is frozen, the more nutrients it retains. Freezing food is also the quickest, easiest, and safest procedure of all the techniques for preserving. Vegetables are simply blanched, cooled, packaged, and frozen. Fruit is cut, dipped in an ascorbic acid bath, and frozen, or cooked in a syrup and frozen. Tomato sauces can be made when tomatoes are falling off the vines, and frozen for a ready-made midwinter spaghetti sauce. Lasagna can be made in double batches and frozen for a busy day. By placing food into temperatures of around 0°F, as is found in most freezers, the activity of microorganisms is halted, and the enzyme process is significantly slowed.

Secrets for Success

Freezer burn—the common term for frozen food that has shriveled up and tastes like cardboard—happens because the food has lost its moisture and become dehydrated. You therefore need to package the food you are going to place in the freezer in containers that hold in all the moisture. Any food in a package that is not sealed properly—aluminum foil with a tear, a freezer bag that isn't closed—will get freezer burn, as will food that is packaged in paper or plastic that does not provide a vapor barrier. Another reason for packaging frozen food in airtight containers is that exposure to oxygen will hasten spoilage. Plastic freezer bags, rigid plastic freezer containers, and glass canning jars all provide a vapor barrier and are airtight.

Freezing food fast is another rule of thumb for successful freezing. Enzymes and microorganisms will continue doing their work until the food is placed in the deep cold of a freezer. Plan ahead so that you don't run out of time to completely process the food, leaving the food to sit overnight, even in the refrigerator. You also need to make sure the freezer maintains its 0°F temperature for a quick freeze. If you add too much food to the freezer at once it will be hard to maintain 0°F. The general rule of thumb is to not add food to a freezer faster than one pound to a cubic foot of freezer space a day.

Most fruits and vegetables have been in liquid before being frozen. If you pack them into a freezer container and freeze them saturated with moisture, they will all freeze together into a lump. This would make it difficult, for example, to separate broccoli flowerets later if you just wanted to take out a few broccoli flowerets at a time. A tip to avoid this problem is to place the broccoli flowerets onto a cookie sheet after blanching and cooling, laying them out so the pieces don't touch one another, and then place them into the freezer for three to four hours. Immediately package the broccoli (it won't stick together), and replace in the freezer.

EQUIPMENT

FREEZER

If you plan to freeze a substantial amount of food, there is no getting around the need for a large-capacity freezer. This one requirement can be an expensive one, but not as expensive as you might think. In the spring of 1996 (the time this chapter is being written), Sears sells a 7.5-cubic-foot upright freezer for three hundred dollars, and a 7.2-cubic-foot chest freezer for the same amount. You can pack a lot of food into freezers this size. The advantage of buying a freezer new is that you will benefit from the advances in energy efficiency. The freezers mentioned above cost only from eight to forty-seven dollars a year to run, depending on how much you are charged per kilowatt hour. Large-capacity freezers are available used for as little as fifty dollars. Older freezers will cost more to run, but you will pay much less up front. (For more on freezers, see chapter 6.)

FREEZER PACKAGING

In choosing freezer packaging, one faces a dilemma about plastic. Other than glass canning jars, the only reliable and easily accessible freezer packaging is made from heavy plastic. It is even recommended to encase heavy-duty aluminum foil in plastic to help seal it, because the foil rips so easily. But, as noted in chapter 2, using plastics is undesirable not only because their use depletes virgin resources, but plastic can also migrate into warm and fatty foods with potential health consequences.

Given the dearth of options, and with a few words of caution, the three packaging options I suggest for harvesting fruits and vegetables are reusable plastic quart freezer containers with snugly fitting lids making an airtight seal, glass canning jars and tops, and plastic freezer bags. The plastic quart freezer containers are made of No. 2 HDPE, and once the containers have finally reached the end of their functional life, in most communities you will be able to recycle them. Glass mason jars come in pint and quart sizes and are available in most hardware stores. They are ideal for homemade sauces such as apple and tomato. Freezer bags come in a variety of sizes, but make sure the labels clearly state that the bags are "freezer" bags, otherwise they may not work as a vapor barrier. Freezer bags are very sturdy, and should be able to be washed and reused a great number of times.

When plastic containers are new, make sure to wash them thoroughly a number of times. The most important thing to remember, however, is never to treat freezer bags as "boil-in-a-bags," and to pack foods after they have cooled. Warm plastic can transfer chemicals to the food.

If you want to freeze casseroles and other food that won't fit in the containers mentioned above (note that freezer bags are available in gallon sizes), use a double layer of heavy-duty aluminum foil. (Make sure that the shiny side is facing the food, as the dull side is coated with an oil.) Seal the package shut by folding the foil and then taping over the fold with tape. Make sure to place food wrapped in foil in a place where it is unlikely to get punctured.

* Label all containers with a grease pencil. Try to avoid indelible ink markers; their solvents linger in the environment and can be toxic, and something written in indelible ink may no longer be appropriate when you want to reuse the container.

Foods Good for Freezing

The sky is virtually the limit when it comes to foods that are good candidates for freezing. In fact, the only limit really is your imagination. While it is not quite true that absolutely everything freezes well (lettuce is out, cucumbers need to be made into a soup, and beans can get mealy), you may be surprised at the variety of foods suitable. Buying eggs on sale can be worth it, for example, because they freeze beautifully by cracking a bunch, blending with a fork, and pouring into ice cube trays. Once frozen, place individual "egg cubes" in a freezer bag for future use. One cube equals an egg. Even dairy products like milk, cream, cottage cheese, and butter can be frozen! Buy food when it is cheap and locally produced, and freeze it for when it is neither.

Freezing Procedure

* As soon as you can after the produce enters your kitchen, prepare it for freezing.
* Wash, peel, slice, core, and cut away bad spots.

FREEZING VEGETABLES

* If you have a double sink and one side has a plug, scrub one sink until it is scrupulously clean and rinse thoroughly. If you don't have a double sink, use a large pan.

Fruits and Vegetables for Freezing

FRUIT

Apples, apricots, avocados, berries, melons, cherries, coconut, currants, figs, grapefruit and oranges, grapes, peaches, nectarines, pears, persimmons, pineapple, plums, prunes, rhubarb, watermelon.

VEGETABLES

Artichokes, asparagus, beans, beets, broccoli, brussels sprouts, cabbage, carrots, cauliflower, celery, collards, corn, eggplant, greens, herbs, kohlrabi, leek, onions, okra, parsnips, peas, peppers, potatoes, pumpkin, rutabagas, soybeans, squash (summer and winter), sweet potatoes, tomatoes, turnips.

* While the vegetables are blanching (see directions earlier in this chapter), fill the cleaned sink or pan with cold water and ice from two or three ice trays.
* Once the vegetables have been blanched the correct amount of time, plunge them, basket and all, into the sink of ice cold water.
* Cool the vegetables thoroughly in the ice water, and then with a slotted spoon remove them and place them on a cookie sheet. (Make sure there is only one layer of vegetables on the sheet, and that the pieces aren't touching each other.) Place immediately in the freezer for three to four hours. Remove and drop into freezer bags or freezer containers, label, and return to the freezer.

FREEZING FRUIT IN SYRUP

The way I freeze pears—freezing fruit in a syrup—is typical of how fruit is usually prepared for freezing. A friend has a few pear trees and gives me bagfuls of pears in October. I line them up in windowsills until they are perfectly ripe, and then I take a few evenings to freeze them, by cutting them into slices, coring them, and cooking with water, honey to taste, and freshly grated ginger root. I cool the mixture, package it in quart freezer containers (meal size), and freeze them. I could have added a bit of lemon juice to make sure the pears didn't brown, but I find I don't need to. Freezing fruit in a sweetened syrup, even if natural sweeteners are used, turns the fruit into a dessert. If you want to avoid the addition of sweeteners, simply freeze the fruit with a compatible fruit juice instead. For freezing fruit without packing it in liquid, see page 190. If packing fruit in a liquid but not a syrup, see page 185 for directions for using an acid-bath pretreatment.

SYRUPS

The general formula for light syrups is:

Light Syrup

½ cup honey to 4 cups water
1 cup sugar or Sucanat to 4 cups water
½ cup maple syrup to 4 cups water

Fruit Juice Syrup

Add fruit and enough fruit juice to cover to a pan. Simmer the fruit until cooked; cool, freeze immediately. (Or, don't cook the juice and fruit, just pack raw.)

Addition of Ascorbic Acid or Lemon Juice

The general formula for the addition of ascorbic acid or lemon juice to syrup is ¼ teaspoon ascorbic acid, or 2 tablespoons lemon juice, per cup of liquid. For a list of fruits appropriate to treat with an acid, please see page 188.

OTHER IDEAS FOR FREEZING FOODS

The freezer is the perfect aid for practicing thrift. Not only can one buy food when it is cheap and freeze it, but you can also significantly reduce the amount of food you waste. For example, if bananas are beginning to get overripe and you don't have time to make banana bread, simply mash up the bananas, add a little lemon juice, and freeze for a time when you can bake. Freezing food is also an incredible asset for establishing a healthful diet in very busy lives. Food can be frozen in advance for days when you know you won't have time to cook, and when you have time and desire to cook, you can make extra of everything for freezing. Here are some other ideas:

* If you enjoy making soup in the winter, keep a large freezer bag of loose vegetables stored in the freezer. Every time you are chopping vegetables, cut a little extra and throw into this all-purpose "soup bag."
* If you like pesto, make a number of batches at once. Spoon it into meal-size yogurt containers, and freeze. (Omit the pine nuts when you do this, and add them just before serving.)
* If you don't use up ginger root very quickly, and tend to throw a lot away because it goes bad, freeze some root in a small freezer bag, take it out and grate off only as much as you need, and replace it in the freezer.
* Make herb "cubes" by cutting up some fresh herbs, placing a teaspoon or so of them in an ice cube tray, covering the herbs with water, and freezing. (You can do this with mint for "mint cubes" for your tea in the winter.)
* To avoid having all of your pans end up in the freezer, buy inexpensive, reusable aluminum pans, available in most supermarkets. Make double batches of casseroles, lasagnas, and favorite dishes, transfer them to the aluminum pans, and freeze.

FINAL STEPS

* Never pack a canning jar, freezer container, or freezer bag completely full. Water expands when it freezes, and the bag would explode.
* Make sure that containers are sealed completely before freezing! This can make the difference between delicious and tasteless food.

* Label and date all food that is put in the freezer.
* As a general guideline, don't refreeze food that has been thawed, especially meat and seafood. Refrozen food loses its flavor, and the food may have become slightly spoiled when it thawed.
* Most fruits and vegetables last up to ten months in a freezer.

DRYING FOOD

The increasing popularity of sun-dried tomatoes has generated interest in drying other foods at home. The flavors of dried foods are very concentrated and are a welcome addition to many dishes.

Moisture is an essential ingredient needed by microorganisms to multiply, and by drying food (removing the moisture) you retard their growth. Once the food is dry it is very lightweight, ideal for camping or travel, and if stored in airtight containers, it will last a long time. Dried vegetables are excellent for soups (peas, zucchinis, carrots, string beans, tomatoes), and dried fruit makes good snacks, and it can be rehydrated to be used in pies and other desserts.

If you live in a climate that is sunny, warm, and dry, you need little more than a drying rack or two to place in the sun. You can't get much easier or cheaper than that! On the other hand, if your climate is more humid, and you want to do a lot of drying, making or buying dehydrating equipment is essential. But if you want to start off slowly and experiment with drying some tomatoes, the oven will be adequate. What is virtually guaranteed is that you will want to dry larger quantities of foods every year. It is very sad indeed when the jar of dried tomatoes is empty by Thanksgiving, with nine long months to go until tomatoes are ripe again.

SECRETS FOR SUCCESS

The three main elements necessary for drying food successfully are heat, air circulation, and time.

HEAT

The USDA recommends a steady drying heat of 140°F. While this is a little higher than some books recommend, mold growth is inhibited at 140°F, an important factor.

TIME

It is important that you don't interrupt the drying process because that could encourage mold growth. Also, the faster the food is dried, the more nutritious it is.

It is difficult to reach 140°F with outdoor drying, but if you choose this method, make sure that you bring the food in at night and place it in a very low oven for the evening, before placing it outside in the sun again the next day. (Make sure to bring the trays in before the dampness of early evening.) Or, if you have an electric food dehydrator, keep the dehydrator going continuously until the food is dried.

AIR CIRCULATION

When food dries, moisture is pulled from the food to its surface, where it evaporates. When there isn't enough air circulation, as can happen with electric dehydrators without fans, or drying in the oven with the oven door closed, moisture clings to the surface of the food, allowing mold to grow.

FOOD-DRYING EQUIPMENT

DRYING RACKS

Unless you buy an electric dehydrator already equipped with drying racks, you will more than likely need to make your own, using the following materials.

    lumber, 1 inch thick by 2 inches wide
    lath

cheesecloth or stainless steel screening (26 inches by 26 inches
  per tray)
staple gun
hammer and nails

1. Make the frame out of ½-inch lumber, or so-called scrap
   lumber (used lumber is fine). A good tray size is 2 feet by
   2 feet. If you are making your own food dehydrator, make
   sure that the tray sizes match what is required for that
   design. Join corners so that they are flush.
2. The cheapest material to stretch over the screen, allowing
   air circulation, is cheesecloth. Stretch it over the entire
   frame and staple to the wood. Prop up the cheesecloth with
   pieces of lath so it doesn't sag in the middle, either crossing
   on the back of the frame (looking like a big X), or placing it
   every ten inches or so. Another choice is stainless steel
   screening. (Do not use the more commonly available galva-
   nized, aluminum, or fiberglass screening because of potential chemical cross-reactions between the food and the
   screen.) Stainless steel screening is hard to find and expensive, but it is well worth it. The following source offers
   stainless steel screening at ten dollars a square foot:
   McMasters Catalog, New Jersey, 908-329-3200.
3. Stretch the screening or cheesecloth over the frame, and
   hold in place with staples or nails.

READY-MADE AND ELECTRIC DEHYDRATORS

Available shaped like a box or round, both versions have trays and
are made with heating coils and sometimes a fan. We don't advise
buying food dehydrators without fans, as the food can more easily
get moldy and spoiled. Make sure that the dehydrator has adequate
ventilation.

OVEN

Make sure to crack the oven door, for air circulation. Also, only use
the oven if you can ensure a temperature of around 140°F, no higher.

OUTDOOR DRYING SHEDS

Drying sheds are fine if you live in a very dry climate, such as the Southwest, but in most of the country outdoor sheds are not very effective because the nights are so damp and dewy that the moisture seeps into the shed, interfering with the drying process.

GENERAL DRYING PROCEDURE

1. Wash, core, and remove stems of produce to be dried. Make sure the fruits and vegetables are ripe.
2. Cut the produce into uniform, thin slices. This is important, as thicker sections will take longer to dry than others, overdrying some parts and underdrying other parts.
3. Blanch vegetables or pretreat fruit, as described earlier in this chapter. (Pretreatment by blanching or treating with an acid is recommended.)
4. Place fruits and vegetables on dryer trays. Lay them in one layer, without overlapping.
5. Start the drying process, be it in the sun, oven, or an electric food dehydrator.
6. If you are using a solar drying method, make sure to remember to bring the food in before dusk, and to place in a warm oven for the night. (A gas stove with a pilot light is enough.)
7. General guidelines for drying times are listed in the table. However, some people like food to be less dried and more pliable (but the food doesn't last as long) than others, so match the drying length to your taste.
8. Make sure to discard any dried food that appears moldy.
9. Dried food lasts for six to nine months.

MAKING FRUIT LEATHERS

Fruit leathers, which are very popular with children, are made by following these steps:

1. Wash, core, and remove stems of produce to be dried. Make sure the fruit and vegetables are ripe.

Drying Fruits and Vegetables

Fruit/veggie	Pretreatment	Cut	Dry Time (in hrs.)*	Doneness
Apples	ascorbic acid	slice	6	suedelike
Asparagus	steam blanch	1 inch slices	2–3	leathery
Apricots	ascorbic acid	slice	14	suedelike
Bananas	none	slice	2–6	brittle
Beans, green	steam blanch	whole/ sliced	3–5	brittle
Beets	cook or steam	slice	3–5	brittle
Berries	none	whole	4	like raisins
Broccoli	steam blanch	florets	3–6	brittle
Brussels sprouts	steam blanch	halve	2–5	brittle
Carrots	steam blanch	slice	3–5	suedelike
Cauliflower	steam blanch	florets	3–6	brittle
Cherries	prick skin	pitted	6	like raisins
Celery	steam blanch	1-inch slices	2–4	brittle
Corn on cob	steam blanch	whole	2–6	brittle
Corn off cob	steam on cob	cut off cob	1–3	brittle
Dates	none	halve	12	like "dates"
Eggplant	steam blanch	slice	2–5	brittle
Figs	scald	halve	5	like "dates"
Grapes	none	halve/ whole	8	like raisins
Mushrooms	none	slice	4–5	suedelike
Okra	none	halve	4–5	brittle
Onions	none	dice	1–6	brittle
Parsnips	steam blanch	slice	4–6	brittle

*Dry Time is equal to the number of hours in the oven or dehydrator, not in the sun. Double the time for sun drying (not including the night).

Drying Fruits and Vegetables (continued)

Fruit/veggie	Pretreatment	Cut	Dry Time (in hrs.)*	Doneness
Peaches	ascorbic acid	slice	6	suedelike
Pears	ascorbic acid	slice	6	suedelike
Peas	steam blanch	shell/ whole pod	3–4	dry/brittle
Peppers	none	sliced	3–5	brittle
Plums (prunes)	scald	halve	6	prunes
Potatoes	steam blanch	slice	2–6	brittle
Pumpkin	steam blanch	slice	4–6	brittle
Spinach	steam blanch	de- stemmed	2–5	brittle
Squash	steam	slice	2–6	brittle
Sweet potatoes	steam blanch	slice	3–6	suedelike/ brittle
Tomatoes	none	slice	4–8	suedelike
Turnips	steam blanch	slice	3–6	suedelike
Zucchini	steam blanch	slice	2–5	brittle

*Dry Time is equal to the number of hours in the oven or dehydrator, not in the sun. Double the time for sun drying (not including the night).

2. Puree the fruit in a food processor until it has formed a thick paste.
3. Using a spatula, smooth the paste onto an oiled cookie sheet.
4. Dry until it is no longer sticky.

DRYING HERBS

If you grow herbs, or can find them fresh locally, you can easily dry some for use in the winter. As with directions for general drying, above, it is important to dry the herbs quickly to avoid losing flavor and nutritional value.

1. The flavorful oils in leafy herbs such as basil are the strongest just before the plant blossoms, so this is the best time to pick. (Other leafy herbs include marjoram, mint, and savory.)
2. Pick early in the morning, which is when the leaves have the most oils.
3. Using scissors, or pinching between two fingernails, clip off the top of the plant.
4. If the herbs need to be washed, rinse quickly and spin and then air dry.
5. The ideal temperature to dry herbs is 105°F.
6. It is important to dry herbs away from sunlight. The darker the better.
7. The most successful way to dry herbs is to hang them upside down, so that as much oil as possible migrates to the leaves. For this reason, hanging herbs upside down in a warm, dark, dry place, such as in an attic or even an upstairs closet, is ideal.
8. To hang herbs, wrap a string around the stems, tie in a knot, leaving at least twelve to twenty-four inches of string. Get a brown paper bag (this will keep the herbs from getting dusty), punch holes in it (make sure you make a lot of holes for adequate air circulation), and dangle the herbs into the bag, allowing the string to escape the top of the bag. Use the string to tie the bag shut, with a bit remaining to tie to a rafter, nail, hook, or whatever is available.
9. Food dehydrators and ovens, while adequate, do not allow for hang drying. If you use a food dehydrator or oven, try to regulate the temperature to around 105°F, and make sure there is air circulation.
10. Herbs are dry when the leaves easily crumble.

OLD WIVES' TALE?

According to folk legend, herbs' leaves should be gathered when the moon is waning (the two weeks after the full moon), and roots when the moon is waxing (the two weeks before the full moon). Leaves reportedly are easier to dry at this time because they retain less moisture, and roots because they are at their most tender.

Drying Herb Seeds

1. Pick the seed pods once they start turning brown.
2. As with all herbs, pick in the morning.
3. Hang dry, as directed for herbs, inside brown paper bags. Once thoroughly dried, the seeds will fall and be caught by the bag.

How to Store Dried Foods

1. Some people like to give dried food a "hit" of high heat, or plunge it into a freezer, at the very end of the drying process to discourage mold growth. To do this with heat, place the food on drying racks in the oven, at 175°F, for just ten or fifteen minutes. For the freezer, place the dried food in freezer bags or containers, and freeze for two or three days.
2. Place dried food in airtight containers (glass jars with screw tops are ideal), and store it away from light, such as in a dark cabinet or closet.
3. The ideal temperature for storage should be a cool room temperature, of around 60°F.
4. Check the stored food every week or so, and give it a shake. If moisture condensation has developed, return the food to the drying process right away.
5. You can freeze food that has been dried by placing it in an appropriate freezer container (see page 191) and placing in the freezer.

Rehydrating

You can use dried food as is, or you can return moisture to the food to soften it and make it pliable. To rehydrate, place the dried fruits or vegetables in a bowl and cover with cold water. Once the food is soft enough for your taste or use (the longer it soaks, the softer it gets), remove and use as you would the equivalent fresh food.

ROOT CELLARS

I think of my root cellar as a secret underground garden into which I spirit away many of my crops when winter threatens.

—Eliot Coleman, author of *The New Organic Grower's Four-Season Harvest*

Root cellars retard the growth of microorganisms and slow down the growth of enzymes by storing food at a very cool (32°F to 40°F) temperature. If you live in a climate where the temperature hovers around freezing or below in the winter, you may want to consider establishing a root cellar for yourself. In fact, if you live in an old house, you may already have one in your basement. They are typically small rooms built into the northwest corner—the coldest spot—of the basement. And there are a number of creative ways to establish or build root cellars that are very inexpensive. The enclosed steps leading down into the basement from a bulkhead entrance can be an ideal place for storing some food, for example, and using that space will cost nothing. The great thing about a root cellar is being able to buy or grow bushels of fresh fruit and vegetables, and keep them crisp and fresh well into the winter. There is nothing like having a plentiful supply of apples, potatoes, onions, pears, garlic, sweet potatoes, and more.

TEMPERATURE

Correct temperature is crucial in establishing a successful root cellar. A root cellar is colder than a refrigerator (temperatures average between 40°F to 50°F). Many of the foods, such as apples, need to be at 32°F to 35°F to retain their crispness. Obtaining *and maintain-*

ing the right temperature can take some work. As you read below about the different types of root cellar structure, think about where the coldest spots are in and around your house, and how they can be modified to create ideal root cellar conditions. For example, I want to build a root cellar in my house (I live in upstate New York) and spent some time leaving a thermometer in different spots around the basement in the middle of the winter. While there is an oil burner down there, the basement isn't heated, and one corner maintains about a 45°F temperature. Hmmmm. If we built a room there with a small window, insulated the room, placed a thermometer in it and cracked open the window for some cold air occasionally, we would have a good root cellar. Occasionally it could get too cold, I presume, but quick use of a space heater could solve the problem.

Some food, such as sweet potatoes, can be maintained at a higher temperature (50°F to 60°F). Again use a thermometer and place it in likely spots. The top of the basement stairs in my house, for example, is about 50°F in the winter, so that is an ideal spot to place a bin for sweet potatoes. (See the table on page 208 to determine the ideal root cellar temperatures for different foods.)

Moisture

If there is not enough moisture in the root cellar, the food will get dehydrated, shrivel up, and become ruined. In fact, for most foods, the humidity in a root cellar has to be really high, between 80 to 90 percent—virtually a rain forest! To create this high humidity, many people place pans of water on the floor of the root cellar. At the hardware store you can buy a humidistat (about an eight-dollar investment) to help monitor the moisture.

Equipment

    Thermometer
    Humidistat
    Bins, crates, baskets

Types of Root Cellars

BASEMENT ROOT CELLAR

The ideal root cellar is an eight-by-ten-foot insulated room, with a window that opens to the outdoors and a dirt floor, in the northwest corner of an unheated basement. This is ideal because the insulation will hold the temperature quite steady, the window will allow ventilation and make cold air accessible if needed, and it is large enough to hold a lot of food. Also, the northwest corner insures no direct sunlight, and the dirt floor insures moisture!

Consult with or hire a builder if you want to add a root cellar to your basement. If you don't have a dirt floor, place pans of water on the floor as needed. Make sure that the door fits tightly, and that there is a lightbulb in the room. When the room has been built, build shelves for food storage. (Place the food that likes warmer temperatures on the highest shelves.)

UNHEATED GARAGE ROOT CELLAR

If you have a garage that is large enough to add a small room, it could be a perfect space for a root cellar. Make sure the root cellar does not get direct sunlight.

GARDEN PIT ROOT CELLARS

Most books on root cellars talk about digging a pit in the garden to use as a root cellar. People apparently place food in pipes and even refrigerators that they then submerge in the pit. The theory is that the earth will insulate the containers in the pit, helping to maintain a steady temperature. Well, I have some very industrious neighbors who have tried every conceivable pit-type root cellar and they claim that water gets into the food no matter what, and that the food also freezes and is defrosted over and over again, ruining it. In other words, don't get your hopes up that the pit-type root cellar will work very well.

For more on making your own root cellar, consult resources for this chapter.

"KEEPERS"

Ever heard of a keeper potato? "Keepers" are long-lasting varieties of different fruits and vegetables, and a detail to pay attention to if you are planning a root cellar of your own. Ask farmers for some varieties of fruit and potatoes that keep the longest.

ROOT CELLAR PROCEDURE

1. Pick or choose the produce when it is as ripe as possible, depending on frosts.
2. Break off leaves, such as carrot tops.
3. Make sure that the produce hasn't been damaged.
4. Some vegetables should be "cured" (allowed to be out in warm, open air to develop a tough outer skin) before they are placed in a root cellar. An easy rule of thumb for determining which vegetables should be "cured" is to think of the ones that will last awhile on your countertop—potatoes, onions, sweet potatoes, garlic, onions, pumpkins, winter squash—and leave those in a warm, sunny environment for a week or two (except potatoes and garlic; keep them in the shade).
5. Do not store fruits and vegetables, or different types of fruit or vegetables, in the same bins, bags, or other containers.
6. Since heat rises, place the food that likes the warmest temperatures highest.
7. Check produce frequently and remove anything that is rotten.

CANNING FOOD

Canning works to preserve food by deactivating enzymes and killing microorganisms. It does this by heating the foods to a very high heat for a specific length of time. Once canned at the right temperature, the containers are airtight, ensuring no further contamination. Food for canning is divided into two groups, low-acid and high-acid. The low-acid foods *must* be heated to 240°F to kill

Root Cellar Storage Details

Fruit/ Vegetable	Humidity	Storage Time (mos.)	Ideal Temperature (°F)
Apples	high	4–6	32–35
Beets	high	4–6	32–40
Broccoli	high	1–2	32–40
Brussels sprouts	high	1–2	32–40
Cabbage	med/high	2–4	32–35
Carrots	high	6–8	32–40
Cauliflower	high	1–2	32–40
Celery	high	6–8	32–35
Chinese cabbage	high	2–4	32–35
Endive, escarole	med/high	2–3	32–35
Garlic	med/dry	6–8	35–40
Grapefruit	med/high	1–2	32–35
Grapes	med/high	1–2	32–35
Horseradish	high	4–6	32–35
Jerusalem artichokes	high	1–2	32–40
Kohlrabi	high	2–3	32–40
Leeks	high	2–4	32–35
Melons	med/high	1–2	40–50
Onions	med/dry	4–6	35–40
Oranges	med/high	1–2	32–35
Parsnips	high	4–6	32–35
Pears	high	2–3	32–35
Peppers, hot	med/dry	4–6	50–60
Potatoes, sweet	med/dry	3–5	50–60
Potatoes, white	med/high	4–6	35–40

Root Cellar Storage Details (continued)

Fruit/ Vegetable	Humidity	Storage Time (mos.)	Ideal Temperature(°F)
Pumpkins	med/dry	4–6	50–60
Rutabagas	high	2–4	32–35
Squash, winter	med/dry	4–6	50–60
Tomatoes, green	med/dry	4–6	50–70
Turnips	high	2–4	32–35
Winter radishes	high	32–35	

med/dry=60–67 percent humidity

med/high=80–90 percent humidity

high=90–95 percent humidity

C. botulinum, whereas the high-acid foods can be heated to 212°F and still be safe. As you will see, sometimes tomatoes fall in the middle, such as the new low-acid variety, and these must be handled in a special way.

Some people are wary of canning for fear of the deadly *C. botulinum,* the bacterium that grows in canned foods and causes the often fatal illness botulism. The rare cases of botulism occur when people can food improperly (they don't follow modern guidelines with modern equipment), not because there is a random chance that home-canned food will have *C. botulinum.* There is a big difference. Acidic foods have a much lower possibility of ever having *C. botulinum* because the bacterium finds acids to be a hostile environment. Armed with this knowledge, we can with confidence learn to can. Making home-canned tomatoes, salsa, and pickles to last through the winter would be a fabulous treat.

BOTULISM

C. botulinum is a bacterium that grows in soil, so it is therefore commonly found on plants. It becomes a deadly poison as it develops spores, which cause the illness botulism. The bacterium thrives in the exact conditions found inside a container of canned food: room temperature, no oxygen, and a lot of moisture. *C. botulinum* has no smell and does not indicate its presence in any other way. It is killed at high heat—240°F. Canning directions are made precisely to kill *C. botulinum,* so if you follow every procedure exactly, there should be no risk.

ACIDITY OF FOODS

As mentioned above, knowing the acidity of foods is critical for safe canning.

Any food with a pH of or below 4.6 (high-acid foods) needs to be heated to a temperature of 212°F for a length of time specific to that food in a boiling water canner (see "Equipment," page 211). Any food with a pH above 4.6 (low-acid foods) must be heated to a temperature of 240°F in nothing other than a pressure canner.

LOW-ACID FOODS (pH ABOVE 4.6)

Pumpkins, carrots, beets, squash, beans, spinach, cabbage, turnips, peppers, sweet potatoes, asparagus, potatoes, mushrooms, peas, corn.
    Required Equipment: Pressure canner only.

HIGH-ACID FOODS (pH BELOW 4.6)

Citrus fruit, plums, apples, strawberries, rhubarb, berries, cherries, peaches, apricots, pears, pineapple, tomatoes (see below for more on tomatoes).
    Required Equipment: Boiling water canner or pressure canner.

TOMATOES: A SPECIAL CASE

Not all tomatoes have a pH below 4.6. In recent years low-acid varieties have been developed that can push the pH above 4.6, into the low-acid category.
    Required Equipment: You must increase the acid content of low-acid tomatoes if you want to use a boiling water canner. In fact, you

should do this as a matter of course for any tomatoes to be processed in a boiling water canner. The Cornell Cooperative Extension Service recommends adding two tablespoons of bottled lemon juice per quart of tomatoes. For pints, use one tablespoon of bottled lemon juice. You can use a pressure canner without adding the extra acid.

Note: Bottled lemon juice is recommended instead of freshly squeezed because it has a consistent acidity.

EQUIPMENT

* Pint and quart canning jars, lids, and rubber rings (if required)

   Note: If the jars you use require rubber rings, you must use new rings every time. Used rings may have lost their ability to make a perfect seal. Also, you must use jars designed for canning so that the glass is thick enough to withstand the high heat of the canners.

* Spoons, ladles, slotted spoons, colander
* Knives, vegetable peelers, corers, etc.
* Funnels
* Jar gripper
* Accurate timer for small amounts of time such as a minute or two
* Canners

   * *Boiling Water Canners:* These canners are usually enamel and come with a wire rack insert to hold the jars in place, and a cover. The canner needs to be deep enough for water completely to cover quart jars, leaving room at the top to hold in rapidly boiling water. (When you are in the store to buy a boiling water canner, it is worth placing a quart jar in the canner to make sure there is enough headroom.) Pressure canners will do, just leave off the tops.
   * *Pressure Canners:* Do not confuse a pressure canner with a pressure cooker. Pressure canners are especially made for processing foods with steam and are equipped with

a safety valve and a petcock opening. They usually cost from $100 to $250. Pressure canners are becoming more and more difficult to find every year, unfortunately. Let your fingers do the walking through the yellow pages, and keep trying until you find a store that sells one. For mail-order catalogs, see "Resources."

PREPARATION FOR CANNING

1. It is critically important that your cutting board, sink, and all equipment be scrupulously clean.
2. Make sure that jars and canners are in perfect working order.
3. Wash lids and rings according to manufacturer's instructions. The two-piece lids are recommended for ease of use and because they have an easily identifiable metal section that will pop up when not sealed properly.
4. Sterilize the jars and a metal knife by placing them in a large container with enough water to cover, bringing to a hard boil, and boiling for fifteen minutes. Leave jars in the hot water until ready to fill (if you add hot food to cold jars the jars can crack).
5. Work as fast as you can. The faster the process is completed, the less chance of any new contamination with microorganisms.

PREPARING FOOD

No matter what kind of food you are canning (high- or low-acid), it is packed either hot or cold in jars, and in a liquid. These two choices are called "hot packs" (the food is placed in the jars cooked and hot, and hot juice, water, or a syrup is poured over it), or "raw packs" (the food is placed in the canning jar without being cooked and is covered with boiling juice or water). If you cook a food for canning, don't let it cool before packing.

Boiling Water Canner: Fruits and Pickles

1. Fill the boiling water canner with enough water to clear the tops of the jars by at least one inch. Turn the heat on high; heat to 180°F.
2. Wash produce thoroughly.
3. Peel, core, slice, or otherwise prepare as appropriate the food for canning.
4. Treat apples, cherries, peaches, or pears with acid treatment as described earlier in this chapter. Let them soak for ten minutes. Remove with a slotted spoon.
5. Have a kettle on the stove ready with boiling water to replenish the water in the pan when needed. If you add cold water the jars will crack.

PACKING LIQUIDS

Note: You will need up to a cup of liquid to pack a quart jar.

For Fruit

Water
Bring to a boil before packing.

Juice
If the fruit is juicy and being hot packed, you may get enough juice from the cooking process, with maybe the addition of a little water, to cover the fruit once it is packed in the jars. If not, use store-bought juice diluted to taste (a lot of varieties of juice are available), or make your own by simmering fruit with a small amount of water, straining off the fruit when soft and mushy, and packing with the liquid. Before packing, heat juice to just boiling.

Syrup
Syrups are virtually synonymous with sweeteners. Heavy syrups are very, very sweet (a one-to-one ratio between sweetener and liquid), and thin syrups are less so (a one-to-three ratio between sweetener and liquid). For the purposes of meeting the goals of the New

Light Syrup

BASIC FORMULA

1 cup sugar	3 cups water/fruit juice

VARIATIONS*

¾ cup honey	3 cups water/fruit juice
½ cup sorghum	3 cups water/fruit juice
¾ cup Sucanat	3 cups water/fruit juice
1 cup maple syrup	3 cups water/fruit juice

*Mix to your taste. Some of the whole food sweeteners can be quite strong in flavor and you may choose to dilute them even more with water or fruit juice. For a lighter syrup add up to 6 cups water/fruit juice.

Green Diet, we will eliminate medium and heavy syrups from our choices. And for thin syrups we suggest substituting whole food sweeteners for refined white sugar. Combine sweetener and liquid in a pan and slowly bring to a boil. Simmer at a low boil for six minutes, stirring constantly.

For Pickles

Pickles and relish require more elaborate preparation than do fruits and vegetables. The following is a good example of a typical pickle recipe. For more recipes for pickles, look up some of the book recommendations under this chapter's resources, or call your cooperative extension.

Ba's Bread and Butter Pickles

> 6 quarts thin, horizontally sliced pickling cucumbers
> 6 medium onions, thinly sliced
> ½ cup pickling salt
> ice cubes
> 1½ quarts white vinegar
> 4½ cups Sucanat

½ cup whole mustard seed
1 tablespoon celery seed
2 tablespoons pickling spice, wrapped in cheesecloth
8 pint jars, or 4 quart jars

a. Put the cucumbers, onions, and salt in a large enamel pot. Stir to combine well. Cover with ice and let sit overnight.

b. Drain the contents of the pot in a colander and in several changes of water. Rinse well.

c. In a large enamel or stainless steel pot, combine the vinegar, sugar, mustard seeds, and pickling spice. Bring the mixture to a boil for several minutes and then add the cucumber and onion mixture. Bring just to a low boil and pack in sterilized jars.

d. Process in a boiling water bath (fifteen minutes for pints, or twenty minutes for quarts) with one inch of water covering the tops of the jars.

1. Packing the Jars

   a. Using slotted spoons, funnels, or whatever will work the best, fill the jars with fruit or pickles. Hot packs should be packed loosely, raw packs can be packed tighter.

   b. Pour the liquid over the food, leaving the amount of headroom required, as given in the table on page 218.

   c. Push a sterilized knife down the edges of the jars to remove any air pockets. Remove knife.

   d. With a clean cloth, wipe the tops of the jars to make sure there is no food that could interfere with a perfect seal.

   e. Put tops on the jars securely.

2. Processing the Jars

   a. Place the jars in the canner, making sure they are covered by at least one inch of water. Replace the lid.

   b. Bring the water to a hard boil. Once it is boiling, you should start the timer according to the times recommended in the table. (If you are at a high altitude, call your state agricultural department for adjustments in boiling times.)

   c. If too much water has evaporated, add some from the kettle.

d. When the time is up, remove the jars and place them on racks.

e. Then seal, if the directions for your type of lid require it.

f. Let the jars cool (up to twelve hours or more).

g. Do not retighten lids! If any seals are loose, discard or reprocess from the beginning.

h. After the jars have cooled, test the seal according to manufacturer's instructions.

i. Label jars with date and contents.

PRESSURE CANNER: LOW-ACID VEGETABLES

1. Follow directions under "Preparation for Canning" (page 212).

2. The vast majority of vegetables need to be blanched before being canned. Turn to the "Blanching" section earlier in this chapter (page 185) and follow the directions specific to the vegetable with which you are working. Save the blanching water; it is rich with nutrients and can be used to pack the food in jars.

3. Have a kettle on the stove full of boiling water.

PACKING THE JARS

1. Once the food is blanched, immediately pack in jars. Fill with the blanching water, leaving a half inch of headroom for all vegetables except corn, peas, and lima beans, which need one inch. If you do not have enough blanching water, or you are using the raw pack technique, use boiling water.

2. Push a sterilized knife down the edges of the jars to remove any air pockets. Remove the knife.

3. With a clean cloth, wipe the tops of the jars to make sure there is no food that could interfere with a perfect seal.

4. Put tops on the jars securely.

Canning Procedure for Acid Foods in a Boiling Water Bath

Food	Hot Pack	Raw Pack	Time to Boil (mins. per pint / quart)
Apples	hot pack sliced ½-inch headroom		15p 20q
Apricots	hot pack peel, halve, pit ½-inch headroom		20p 25q
Berries (not strawberries)	hot pack ½-inch headroom	raw pack ½ inch headroom	10p 15q
Cherries	hot pack prick or pit ½-inch headroom	raw pack prick or pit ½-inch headroom	25p 25q
Grapefruit and other citrus		raw pack seed, segment ½-inch headroom	10p 10q
Peaches	hot pack peel, halve, pit ½-inch headroom		20p 25q
Pears	hot pack peeled, halved, or sliced ½-inch headroom		20p 25q

Canning Procedure for Acid Foods in a Boiling Water Bath (continued)

Food	Hot Pack	Raw Pack	Time to Boil (mins. per pint / quart)
Pineapple	hot pack peel, slice		20p
Plums	hot pack prick ½-inch headroom	raw pack prick ½-inch headroom	20p 25q
Rhubarb	hot pack 1-inch slices ½-inch headroom		10p 10q
Tomatoes (packed in water)	hot pack whole, halved, peeled add acid	cold pack whole, halved, peeled add acid	40p 45q
Tomatoes (packed in juice)	hot pack whole, halved, peeled add acid ½-inch headroom	cold pack whole, halved, peeled add acid ½-inch headroom	85p 85q
Pickles			
Dill		cold pack ½-inch headroom	10p 15q
Sweet gherkin	hot pack ½-inch headroom		10p 15q
Bread and butter	hot pack ½-inch headroom		10p

Canning Procedure for Acid Foods in a Boiling Water Bath (continued)

Food	Hot Pack	Raw Pack	Time to Boil (mins. per pint / quart)
Pickle relish	hot pack ½-inch headroom		10p

Note: If you are at a high altitude, make sure to add time (see page 215).

PROCESSING THE JARS IN A PRESSURE CANNER

1. Pour two or three inches of hot water into the pressure canner.
2. Place the jars on the rack.
3. Close the cover of the canner completely. At this time leave the gauge open and do not close the petcock.
4. Heat until steam escapes, then time for ten minutes. (This is preparing the steamer for canning; it is not canning time.)
5. Follow manufacturer's directions for setting the pressure to ten pounds (240°F). If you live at a higher altitude, adjust accordingly.
6. Once the ten pounds has been reached, set the timer for the exact amount of time required for the particular vegetable you are canning (see table).
7. Take the canner off the heat, return pressure to zero, and wait before opening, according to manufacturer's instructions.
8. When the time is up, remove the jars and place them on racks.
    A. Then seal, if the directions for your type of lid require it.
    B. Let the jars cool (up to twelve hours or more).
    C. Do not retighten lids! If the jars are not sealed properly, discard or reprocess from the beginning.
    D. After the jars have cooled, test the seal, according to manufacturer's instructions. Remove any jars that haven't sealed properly and reprocess.
    E. Label jars with date and contents.

Canning Procedure for Low-Acid Vegetables in a Pressure Canner

Vegetable	Treatment*	Time Needed to Boil	
		pints	quarts
Asparagus	blanched	30	40
Beans,lima	blanched;1-inch headroom	40	50
Beans,snap	blanched	20	25
Beets	cook	30	35
Carrots	blanched	25	30
Corn	cut/blanch; 1-inch headroom	85	85
Greens	blanch	70	90
Okra	blanch	30	40
Peas	blanch;1-inch headroom	40	40
Pumpkin	cooked, cubed	55	90
Squash,summer	blanch/sliced	30	40
Squash,winter	cooked,cubed	55	90
Sweet potatoes	cooked,cubed	65	90
Tomatoes	blanch,peel,cut	30	35

*Unless otherwise noted, pack with ½-inch headroom.

STORING CANNED FOODS

The ideal temperature for storing canned foods is around 60°F. Store away from light.

WARNING SIGNS

Do not eat or open any jar of canned food that has leaked, foams, has a bad appearance, or if the metal top is bulging. Once you open it, if the food has a bad smell or if you see signs of mold anywhere, discard. If you must discard a jar of canned food, it is essential that you do so in a way that no person or animal could possibly eat it. Never put it in a compost.

6

The Ecological Kitchen

The word *ecology* comes from the same Greek root as *economy* does: *oikos,* which means house. Economics was originally a study of the family household and its daily operations and maintenance. The idea of the "house" gradually expanded from the family household to a more holistic notion of home in the larger sense of the greater community. It studied how the community as a whole manages its resources. The term *ecology* has a parallel meaning: first coined in 1873 by Ernst Haeckel, a German Darwinian, the term is defined as a study of how organisms interact with one another and their total environment.

Carefully choosing what comes into our kitchen and what goes out of it as waste, according to its effect on ourselves and our environment, is the way to establish our kitchen as an ecological system. All of us bring food, packaging, cleaning products, building materials, energy, appliances, and items for pest control into our homes. Most of us also pour toxic cleaning products down drains, put packaging in landfills and incinerators, throw broken refrigerators full of chlorofluorocarbons (CFCs) into dumps, and the list goes on. All of these activities have impacts on the environment and on our health. We can significantly reduce the amount our own families pollute the environment by monitoring the products we bring into our homes, using them wisely, and disposing of them responsibly.

UNDER THE KITCHEN SINK: HOUSEHOLD HAZARDOUS WASTE

Almost everyone in the United States has a cupboard full of poisons under their kitchen sink. Wasp spray, oven cleaner, waxes and pol-

ishes—the place is full of chemicals that display the words *poison,
danger, warning,* or *caution.* Removing these products from under
the kitchen sink is recommended. Small amounts of the poisons
drift from, and leak out of, bottles and spray bottles, which then
waft around the kitchen. Household poisonings are one of the
highest threats to the health of children. Place products with signal
words in a locked cupboard in an out-of-the-way place such as a
garage. Once you have removed the toxic chemicals, you can make
a fresh start with nonpolluting, biodegradable alternative products.
This chapter will give you plenty of options, so you can bypass
bringing any more hazardous products into your home.

SIGNAL WORDS

The signal words *poison, danger, warning,* or *caution,* found on the
label of products such as pesticides and cleaning products, are
placed there by order of the federal government and are primarily
for your protection. In some cases these signal words are on the
label because of the potential impact the product can have on the
environment. For whatever reason the signal word is on the product, *poison/danger* denotes a product of most concern, one that is
highly toxic, and ingesting small amounts—in some cases a few
drops—can be fatal. *Warning* means moderately toxic, as little as a
teaspoonful can be fatal; and *caution* denotes a product that is less
toxic, one in which it would be necessary to ingest between two
tablespoonfuls and two cups to be fatal. *Extremely flammable/
flammable/combustible* means what it says: the product can catch
fire, so you need to keep it away from any flame. *Corrosive* products
can damage skin and mucous membranes, and a *strong sensitizer* is
a chemical that can increase allergies.

DOWN THE DRAIN

Household hazardous waste should not be thrown into the trash or
poured down the drain. Toxics leach out of landfills and are
released from incinerators, and a polluted stream can pollute our
drinking water. We need to think twice about pouring household

hazardous waste down the drain, even when it is the designated job of the product. One-third of a ton of toilet bowl cleaner is poured down the toilets of an average town of ten thousand *every month*, for example, estimates the Environmental Task Force Vision 2020. Sewage treatment plants have a great deal of work to do to manage this level of toxic chemicals. The chemicals are damaging in home septic systems too, because some of the household cleaners poured down the drain actually kill the bacteria that are necessary for a septic tank to function properly. It is much preferable to use biodegradable products in the home.

CLEANING

Many modern synthetic cleaning products mimic old folk recipes. The reason for this is that the old formulas almost always turn out to be based on good science. Folk recipes for cleaning use natural materials such as the minerals baking soda and washing soda, and acids such as vinegar or lemon juice, all materials that have chemical properties that lend themselves to cleaning.

Using updated versions of the old recipes for cleaning makes it easy to avoid toxic, synthetic cleaning agents. Natural cleaners can be substituted for cleaning products such as furniture polishes and stains, floor waxes, car waxes, spray dust cleaners, drain cleaners, toilet bowl cleaners, oven cleaners, petroleum-based spot and stain removers, all aerosols, and shoe polish.

Learning to clean from scratch by using cleansers made from homemade recipes can truly work if you take time to understand a bit about the chemistry behind how materials such as the mineral baking soda, and acids such as lemon juice, work. Another key to success is to choose the right materials for the right job. The five ingredients that I find to be the safest, most effective, and useful for cleaning are baking soda, washing soda, vinegar and lemon juice, vegetable-oil-based detergents and soaps, and an antifungal essential oil called Australian tea tree oil. Note that ammonia and bleach are not on this list. You don't need them. Make sure to keep all homemade formulas well labeled, and out of the reach of children.

BAKING SODA

This miraculous mineral, sodium bicarbonate, has more uses for household cleaning than any other substance. It is made from soda ash, which is produced from a naturally occurring ore called trona, mined (by deep mining, as opposed to more damaging strip mining) in Wyoming.

Baking soda is slightly alkaline, with a pH around 8.1 (7 is neutral), so it neutralizes acid-based odors in water. Sprinkled on a damp sponge or cloth, baking soda can be used as a gentle cleaner for kitchen countertops. It is also a good scouring powder for sinks and bathtubs and an excellent oven cleanser, and it is gentle enough to be used to clean fiberglass. It will eliminate perspiration odors and even neutralize the smell of many chemicals if you add up to a cup per load to the laundry. If you dislike the "new" smell of new clothes, soak them overnight in water plus a cup of baking soda. The chemical odor will be neutralized.

Baking soda absorbs odors from the air, making it a useful air freshener, as many know from placing an open box of it in the refrigerator. It is also a fine carpet deodorizer: sprinkle it onto carpets and vacuum up an hour later. Last but not least, baking soda can help keep drainpipes clear. When you pour baking soda and boiling water down a drain, you alter the soda's chemical composition, making it more caustic, and thus more effective in breaking down grease and dirt.

WASHING SODA

A chemical neighbor of baking soda, washing soda (sodium carbonate) is more strongly alkaline, with a pH around 11. It is mined much like baking soda but processed differently. Because it is quite caustic, it cannot be called nontoxic, and you should wear rubber gloves when using it. But it releases no harmful fumes and is far safer than a commercial solvent formula.

Washing soda is a real find for natural cleaning because it is a powerful, heavy-duty cleaner. It cuts grease, cleans petroleum oils and dirt, removes wax or lipstick, and softens water. It you have a petroleum spill on the basement or garage floor, washing soda is the cleaner of choice. Washing soda is readily made into scouring powders and soft scrubbers, floor cleaners, and all-purpose cleaners. Traditionally used as a laundry detergent booster, it works well for that job too. It also neutralizes odors in the same way that baking soda does. Washing soda is too caustic to use on fiberglass, aluminum, or waxed floors—unless you intend to remove the wax. For heavy-duty jobs, make washing soda into a thick paste with water, apply, scrub, and rinse well. For less intensive jobs mix one-half to one cup of washing soda per gallon of water. (Warm water is needed to dissolve the washing soda.)

White Vinegar and Lemon Juice

White vinegar and lemon juice are the opposites of baking and washing soda: they are acidic and so neutralize alkaline, or caustic, substances. If your tap water is hard and you have trouble with mineral buildup (scale), soak a cloth in vinegar and rest it on the scale buildup for a few hours. The acid will break down the minerals and they can be wiped away. Acids dissolve gummy buildup and eat away tarnish. I have also found vinegar to be particularly good for removing dirt from wood surfaces.

Liquid Soaps and Detergent

Liquid soaps and detergents are necessary for washing dishes, windows, and floors. Detergents are synthetic materials made up of surfactants (surface active agents), which are derived from vegetable oils, animal fat, or petroleum constituents. Discovered and synthesized early in this century, detergents are considered an improvement over soap because they don't react with hard water minerals. This protects clothes from getting gray and prevents soap scum and film from forming on tiles, tubs, and sinks.

The brands of liquid soaps and detergents that are the purest—without dyes, perfumes, and other additives—are primarily found in health food stores. If you have hard water buy a detergent; if you have soft water you can use a real soap.

DISINFECTANTS

For a substance to be registered by the EPA as a disinfectant, it must go through extensive and expensive tests. There is only one "natural" disinfectant on the market that has been registered by the EPA. It is a hospital-grade disinfectant, achieving a 100 percent kill rate. Called Power Herbal Disinfectant, it is available in health food stores. Australian tea tree oil and grapefruit seed extract are two ingredients that folk legend claims kill bacteria and mold, as well as being successful disinfectants. While not registered with the EPA as disinfectants (although Australian tea tree oil is one of the ingredients in Power Herbal Disinfectant), they do work well for killing mold and mildew. Australian tea tree oil is an essential oil from the melaleuca tree. Australian tea tree oil has a strong but not unpleasant odor that dissipates after a few days. Though this oil is expensive, a little bit goes a long way. A grapefruit seed extract spray can be made by adding twenty drops of extract to a quart of water. Both Australian tea tree oil and grapefruit seed extract are commonly available in health food stores.

CLEANING THE OVEN

Baking soda and water are excellent for cleaning the oven. Sprinkle a cup or more of baking soda over the bottom of the oven, then cover the baking soda with enough water to make a thick paste. Let the mixture set overnight. The next morning the grease will be easy to wipe up because the grime will have been loosened. When you have cleaned up the worst of the mess, dab a bit of liquid detergent or soap on a sponge, and wash the remaining residue from the oven. If this recipe doesn't work for you use more baking soda or water.

CLEANING THE SINK

Simply pour about half a cup of baking soda into a corner of the sink, and slowly add liquid detergent, stirring while you add, until the mixture has a texture like frosting. Scoop the mixture onto a sponge, and wash the sink. Rinse.

Washing the Dishes

The best solution for washing the dishes by hand is to visit a health food store and buy a "green" liquid dish detergent. Health food stores and green supermarkets have a number of brands of liquid dish detergent that are free of perfumes and dyes. What should you use in the automatic dishwasher? Unfortunately there is not yet an environmentally preferable product on the market that works. Even the greenest detergent manufacturers are having trouble coming up with a formula that is effective in hard water and yet isn't made with phosphates. (Phosphates are responsible for algae bloom in the waste-water stream.) While phosphate-free dish detergent may work in areas with soft water, in hard-water areas they tend to coat the dishes with a white film. Keep your eyes out for new product breakthroughs in this area and any advertisements that a product is phosphate-free.

Cleaning Appliances

Start with a clean and empty spray bottle. Add about one-half teaspoon of washing soda, a couple of teaspoons of liquid soap, and two cups of hot tap water. Shake well to dissolve. Variations on this formula can include substituting vinegar (this can double as a window cleaner) or borax for the washing soda.

A wide range of less toxic and biodegradable ready-made commercial cleaning products is increasingly available in health food stores and green supermarkets. The green cleaning product category is highly scrutinized, and the products found in health food stores tend to live up to their claims of being environmentally preferable. Some stores even offer brands in refillable containers. See this chapter's list of resources for more sources of cleaning information.

PEST CONTROL

As discussed in chapter 2, pesticides have many health consequences and their use in and around the home is linked to increased risk of leukemia in children. There are a number of less toxic ways of combating kitchen pests such as ants, flies, and roaches. The best resource of less toxic alternatives is the book *Common Sense Pest Control: Least Toxic Solutions for Your Home, Garden, Pets and Community* (see "Resources"). It is an expensive resource book, but you can suggest your local library get a copy of it as a community service. Another excellent resource is the Rachel Carson Council. They offer a number of publications that are pest-specific, with practical and safe ways to eradicate the pest. (See listing in "Resources.")

ANTS

In a bowl, mix one cup borax, one cup sugar, and three cups water. Place a loose wad of toilet paper into four different screw-top jars that are about the size of shallow marinated artichoke jars. Pour the mixture into the jars until it is about one inch from the top. Screw the lids on the jars, and with a hammer and nail, make four to eight holes in the lid. Place the jars in areas where you have ants, and watch them line up in rows to march in. Keep away from children.

FLIES

Keep the kitchen clean with food put away. Screens are essential to keeping flies out. Fly swatters and flypaper—those sticky spiral bands of paper that hang from ceilings—are adequate for minor fly invasions. *Make sure flypaper is not impregnated with any kind of toxic pesticide,* and that it is kept away from children. The flypaper may include a fly sex attractant (a pheromone), but it is odorless and harmless to humans.

To get rid of household flies in Puerto Rico people hang a plastic bag full of water from a window or a door. The fly sees itself reflected on the bag, but magnified, and flies away in fear!

If you have a serious fly infestation, make a citrus peel spray by simmering six to eight citrus rinds in one to two quarts of water, in a pot on low for two to three hours, refilling as it evaporates. Cool, strain into a spray bottle, and spray areas of infestation. (*Note:* The citrus extract may stain cloth curtains, so test such applications first.) Keep citrus peel spray away from cats.

COCKROACHES

Boric acid is a material derived from borax and has a low toxicity for humans. Available in hardware stores, boric acid powder works effectively to kill cockroaches. It can be put in floor cracks and in many hard-to-reach areas. Just make sure that the white powder cannot be ingested by pets or children. Cockroaches are not repelled by boric acid, as they are by other poisons, so they are more likely to ingest it. It can take five to ten days for the boric acid to kill the roaches. If you have cockroaches, make sure that you have a can or bucket with a secure top for kitchen food scraps. Seal any cracks (where cockroaches love to live) in the walls and floors, and eliminate water sources by fixing leaky plumbing, leaving the sink empty, and pouring out pets' water bowls at night, etc.

GRANARY WEEVILS

As discussed in chapter 4, granary weevils—grain moths—are repelled by bay leaves. Tape the leaves onto the top of cereal and rice boxes, or place inside canisters of flour and other grains.

PROFESSIONAL PEST CONTROL

If you have an infestation that you believe requires professional pest control, choose the company with care. Contact the Rachel Carson Council for their free (with a self-addressed, stamped envelope) "Questionnaire for Interviewing Pest Control Specialists." Least toxic alternatives used by a professional could include special applications of diatomaceous earth, silica aerogel, or boric acid, nematodes that eat termites, heat treatments, and electric currents applied with a gun-type device.

WATER

It is estimated that we waste 20 to 35 percent of the water we use in our homes.

—G. Tyler Miller, *Living in the Environment*

Only 3 percent of the earth's water is fresh, and more than two-thirds of this is frozen in glaciers and polar ice caps. A World Bank study predicts a severe water crisis around the globe over the next decade or two, because of population growth, water contamination, and government subsidies that make water cheap, which can encourage waste.

There are two kinds of drinking water: surface water and groundwater. Surface water is renewable; it comes to us from melting snows, rainwater, runoff, rivers, and streams. Water that is piped to a town from a reservoir, for example, is surface water, as is that pumped in from rivers. During droughts reservoirs get low, as do rivers, and water conservation is critical. One should not tip the scales by using more water than can be replenished. The pollution of surface water is a critical problem. Much of the world population's water comes from rivers, where sewage and factory effluent are dumped.

Groundwater comes from within the earth, where rainwater has seeped down through sand and rock, settling in pores and crevices over a span of hundreds of years. Often pooling in aquifers, groundwater supplies wells and springs. The water table is the upper limit of groundwater, where it can "spring feed" a river or lake. Ultimately groundwater is renewable, but only over a span of many years, not a season, as is the case of surface water. Contamination of groundwater by agricultural pesticides and industrial pollutants is of concern, as the chemicals leach down to the groundwater and migrate into underground rivers. An artesian well that reaches deep into the earth to draw out groundwater can pull up water that has been polluted miles away. According to *Groundwater Pollution News,* roughly 51 percent of the United States population relies on groundwater for some drinking water.

Conserving water and adding as little pollution to it as possible are skills we all need to learn and practice, no matter where we live. Fifty-seven percent of municipally supplied water is to households, so our water use has a big impact.

THE KITCHEN FAUCET

Most of us run the water in the kitchen to flush lead from the pipes (three to five minutes every morning) or until it gets cold or hot, for example. If you buy three or four water pitchers to catch this wasted water every day, to use later for rinsing and washing dishes, or vegetables, or to place in the refrigerator for a source of cold water (but not for cooking or drinking), you can conserve many gallons of water a day. Visit a kitchen store, or look through a kitchen equipment catalog, for a wide variety of attractive water pitcher choices. You can always, of course, use a bucket or pot as well. Keep it under the sink and bring it out to place under the faucet every time you run water that can be used for other purposes such as cleaning or watering plants.

If your kitchen faucet drips, you can waste seventy-five gallons of water a week. By all means have the leak fixed; call a plumber if you can't fix it yourself.

There is a special faucet gadget that can cut water use in half or more. Called an aerator, this inexpensive faucet attachment mixes air into the water as it leaves the tap. While not affecting the volume or pressure, the aerator can reduce a water flow of four to five gallons a minute to two and a half gallons a minute. Some aerators swivel easily in any direction, so you can reach every corner of your sink. Faucet aerators are available from Seventh Generation and Real Goods catalogs (see "Resources").

Faucets can be sources of lead, cadmium, mercury, and other toxic substances. The EPA, the plumbing industry, and public health officials have recently developed standards for how much lead and other toxics a faucet can contribute to the water. Six manufacturers have passed the tests. (Passing means that lead can contribute no more than eleven parts per billion to the lead content of the water.) Look for the NSF International logo on boxes of faucets when you buy them. NSF International is the company that carried out the tests, and you can call them at 800-678-8010 for a full list of approved faucets.

WASHING THE DISHES

The average number of gallons used to wash dishes by hand is fifteen to twenty-five gallons. You can save five gallons of water or so from this process, according to David Goldbeck in *The Smart Kitchen,* by "ponding" water. To pond for hand-washing dishes, fill the sink with water, and wash the dishes in the full sink, instead of washing the dishes under a stream of water. If you have side-by-side sinks, fill both sides with water, wash in one and rinse in the other.

AUTOMATIC DISHWASHERS

A study at Ohio State University found that an automatic dishwasher consumes about 5.8 fewer gallons of water per load than washing the same dishes by hand. While hand-washing uses about 15.7 gallons, the average dishwasher uses 9.9 gallons. If you "pond" the water for hand-washing, the amount of water used can be about the same. To save the most water when using automatic dishwashers, only run when full, rinse food as little as possible, and use the "air-dry" cycle.

GARBAGE DISPOSALS

Garbage disposals use up about two to seven gallons of water per minute, according to April Moore in *The Earth and You, Eating for Two.* Only run when full. Composting is a more ecological choice for food waste.

GRAY WATER

Gray water is all used household water from showers and sinks, never including that which comes from toilets. Most experts recommend against the kitchen sink as a source of gray water because so much oil and bacteria are poured down the kitchen drains. Gray water is no longer recommended to use in vegetable gardens because of the bacteria gray water may contain. If you want to pursue using gray water, contact Metamorphic Press (see "Resources").

CLEAN WATER

As mentioned in chapter 2, an estimated fourteen million Americans drink water contaminated with herbicides, according to a study by the Environmental Working Group. There are also other sources of contamination. Lead and other metals can leach from fixtures, for example. Bacteria and viruses from sewage can seep into wells. According to a report in *Water Technology* magazine, widespread water contaminants include aluminum oxide, atrazine, ethylene dibromide, heavy metals, household cleaners, industrial nonhazardous wastes, nitrates, pesticides, volatile organic compounds, and the prolific pest zebra mussels.

If you are on a municipal water system, law requires that water be disinfected with chlorine. Under the Safe Drinking Water Act of 1974, and with subsequent updates, your municipality must now regularly test for eighty-three possible contaminants. Some contaminants are not tested, and many people wish to remove the taste of chlorine from their water. Filtering water in our homes is increasingly desirable no matter where you may live in America.

Buying springwater in plastic gallon jugs is not the answer for an ecological kitchen, however. Buying a three-hundred-dollar whole house water filter is cheaper by half than the yearly cost of the equivalent amount of water in plastic jugs. And plastic jugs cost the environment dearly, even if they are recyclable in your community, and plastics can leach into the water, contaminating it.

Before buying a water filter you should have your water tested. (Some people on municipal water choose to get just a filter for chlorine and don't test the water.) This will ensure that you can make an educated decision about what kind of water filter to buy, if you need one. Make sure to spend the money to test for a full range of chemicals, such as pesticides and herbicides, however, or you will not be getting a full picture of the safety of your water. If the lead levels in your home's water are above 15 ppb in "first-draw" water—that is, water taken directly from the pipes first thing in the morning—or 5 ppb from flushed pipes, you should invest in a filter, as should you if other chemicals are found in your water even at low levels. Better safe than sorry. Following is a description of the three main kinds of water filters currently available. Each has its good and bad points; unfortunately none is perfect.

CARBON FILTERS

Activated carbon filters are the most common filters on the market. They work to purify water because they absorb contaminants, and as the water passes through the carbon, suspended solids are filtered and trapped by the carbon. Carbon filters can reduce chlorine, some man-made chemicals including chlordane, benzene, and carbon tetrachloride, and some reduce lead. Carbon filters are available in sizes and styles that range from whole house treatment to small pour-through pitchers. Carbon filter cartridges need to be replaced regularly.

Alert: Carbon filters will not remove bacteria or viruses. Some experts recommend carbon filters only be used on municipal water supplies that are continually disinfected with chlorine. Silver-impregnated carbon filters slow the growth of bacteria but do not kill bacteria already in the water.

REVERSE OSMOSIS

In reverse osmosis, water is filtered first through a cartridge that removes suspended solids and then through a membrane that can reduce heavy metals such as lead, mercury, and arsenic, bacteria and viruses, and pesticides and herbicides.

Alert: In reverse osmosis the water comes in contact with a lot of plastic, and some people complain that at first the water tastes of plastic. Also, for each gallon of purified drinking water, you will waste four gallons of water. While this is wasteful enough, systems that do not have shut-off valves continue to waste water when the storage tank is full. Most contemporary reverse osmosis systems have a shut-off valve, but make extra sure before you buy one.

DISTILLATION

Distillers produce the purest water—in fact, it is so pure, all its health-promoting minerals have been removed too. However, the trade-off is that this system reduces chemicals, heavy metals, and bacteria and viruses by 90 percent or more. Distillers work by boiling water, turning it into steam, and cooling it again to a liquid state. Contaminants are left behind in the steam or boiling tank. Most distillers also contain a carbon filter to reduce any volatile organic chemicals present that may not be reduced in the distiller's boiling or steam stage because their boiling point is similar to water.

Alert: While very effective at reducing contaminants, distillers require a lot of electricity to operate. Water-cooled distillers require extra water compared to air-cooled distillers. Choose distillers made of stainless steel, not aluminum, since small amounts of aluminum may leach into the water with unknown health effects. Last but not least, distillers reduce vital minerals such as magnesium from the water supply, and while water is not the only source of these minerals, one needs to make sure to eat a healthful diet to make up for their loss in drinking water.

ENERGY USE IN THE KITCHEN

Some 20 to 40 percent of household energy is consumed in the kitchen.

—David Goldbeck, *The Smart Kitchen*

According to the American Council for an Energy-Efficient Economy's book *Consumer Guide to Home Energy Savings*—a must read for anyone considering buying large appliances—

Every kilowatt-hour (kWh) of electricity you avoid using saves over two pounds of carbon dioxide that would otherwise be pumped into the atmosphere. Carbon dioxide (CO_2) is the number-one contributor to

global warming. . . . If you replace a typical 1973, 18-cubic-foot refrig-
erator with an energy-efficient 1994 model, you'll save over 1,000 kWh
and over a ton of CO_2 emissions per year.

There is a lot at stake in our use of kitchen appliances.

If you are in the market for a new kitchen appliance you also need to be aware of EnergyGuide labels, which are required by federal law to be placed on most new kitchen appliances. Each label will offer you information about who manufactured the product and details such as its model number, how the model compares in energy efficiency to other comparable models, and estimated energy consumption in kWh/year and estimated annual energy costs. If you already have kitchen appliances, there are specific energy-efficiency tips for maintaining them, listed below.

SMALL APPLIANCES

A green kitchen cluttered with small appliances seems a contradiction in terms, yet in terms of energy use alone, small appliances use less energy for specialized cooking jobs than big electric appliances. Baking four potatoes in a toaster oven makes more sense from an energy standpoint than baking the potatoes in a full-size oven, for example. An electric teapot takes less energy than heating a teakettle on the stove, as does using a rice cooker, a crock pot, or an electric fry pan. The reason for this is that the heating element is built right into the small appliance and transfers the heat more efficiently. Microwaves are extremely energy efficient because the source of energy is from electromagnetic waves, not heat. Instead of being consumer indulgences, small appliances are energy savers.

REFRIGERATORS AND FREEZERS

These appliances are the biggest energy users in the kitchen. If you have an old refrigerator it will be worth your while in energy savings to buy a new one. Up-to-date refrigerators are significantly more energy efficient than their older counterparts, saving up to 50 percent in energy costs. Here are some guidelines to help in choosing and maintaining energy-efficient refrigerators and freezers.

* Side-by-side refrigerator/freezers use up to 13 percent more energy than a typical refrigerator with the freezer above or below it.
* Automatic ice makers increase energy use substantially.
* On old refrigerators, manual defrost is the most energy efficient. The automatic defrost on many modern refrigerators, however, is operated by computer chip, and such refrigerators are equal in energy use to the manual defrost counterpart.
* Try not to buy refrigerators with antisweat boosters. Sometimes called a "power-saver switch," they often can be turned off.
* Once a year or more clean the condenser coils found at the back or underside of the refrigerator.
* The ideal temperature for a refrigerator is 38°F to 40°F; 0°F to 5°F for a freezer. Place a thermometer inside the refrigerator to monitor the temperature.
* Make sure that the door gaskets are not ripped or broken in any way.
* Try to place a chest freezer in as cool a room as possible.
* Chest freezers are more energy efficient than uprights because less warm air enters when it is opened.
* Keep the top of the refrigerator uncluttered.
* The fuller a freezer, the more energy efficient.
* Don't place hot foods in the refrigerator or freezer. Cool them to room temperature first.
* Open the doors of refrigerators or freezers as little as possible.
* Make sure the refrigerator or freezer is not in the direct sun, or next to the stove.

DISHWASHERS

Eighty percent of the cost of running a dishwasher is in heating the water, reports David Goldbeck in *The Smart Kitchen*. But as with refrigerators there are ways to reduce the amount of energy consumption.

* The hot water used for dishwashers needs to reach 140°F to remove grease and dissolve detergent. In older dishwasher models the hot water heater for the whole house has to be set at that high temperature, which is very costly in energy use, and unsafe for children as well (they can easily get scalded). Most new dishwashers, however, have a special booster heater to heat the water for the dishwasher alone to the specified 140°F, making it possible to keep the temperature of the house's hot water heater at 120°F instead.
* New models of dishwashers have an air-dry option. Use that whenever possible instead of heat drying. Better yet, open the door of the dishwasher for that last drying cycle.
* Use the shortest dishwashing cycle.
* Only run a full load.
* Try to rinse the dishes as little as possible before stacking in the dishwasher.

STOVES

There are a lot of different options for stoves. Here are some guidelines about how these choices affect your home's energy use.

* Induction cook tops are the most energy efficient. (These are the kind where there is a ceramic cooking surface, looking almost like a countertop.) Almost no heat is wasted beyond the edge of the pan, and the heating stops immediately when the pan is removed.
* Convection ovens are the most energy efficient because heated air is continuously circulated.
* Gas stoves are more energy efficient than electric; however, they cause indoor air pollution. New gas stoves with electronic ignition use around 30 percent less gas than those with a pilot light. Upgrade to an electronic ignition model if you can. To make sure a gas stove is working efficiently, check the flame. It should be bluish. If it is yellow, call the gas company to have the stove adjusted.

COOKING TIPS TO SAVE ENERGY

* Match the size of the pan to the size of the heating coil on ranges.
* Cover pans when cooking.
* Turn off the burner or oven before the food is completely cooked.
* Low-fat and low-liquid cooking lessens cooking time.
* Reheat leftovers on the top of the range instead of in the oven.
* Use a pressure cooker whenever possible.
* Make more food than you need, and freeze the rest for your own "fast food."
* Make a solar box cooker (see information in "Resources").
* Enjoy cooking in one pot. This minimizes both the stove's and your energy expenditure.
* If you eat a lot of pasta, cook a week's worth at once, toss lightly in oil, and keep in the refrigerator.

LIGHTING

A single compact fluorescent lamp . . . can save enough coal-fired electricity over its lifetime to keep a power plant from emitting three-quarters of a ton of carbon dioxide (which contributes to global warming) and fifteen pounds of sulfur dioxide (which causes acid rain).

—Amory and Hunter Lovins in the foreword to
Homemade Money

The Rocky Mountain Institute has compared the total life cycle costs of regular incandescent bulbs and compact fluorescents over ten thousand hours. The total savings from one compact fluorescent is $37.06; the total life cycle cost for 10,000 hours of light with incandescent bulbs is $72, the life cycle cost for the equivalent compact fluorescent light is $34.94. Though more expensive to begin with, using compact fluorescents is a real savings in the long run. Compact fluorescents are available for every kind of fixture and are available in most hardware stores.

PHANTOM LOADS

A phantom load is the cost of maintaining a clock on appliances when not in use, such as coffeemakers, microwaves, and stoves. These phantom loads add up in electrical use. *Home Power* magazine estimates that such "phantom loads" in the United States equal the electricity use of Greece, Peru, and Vietnam combined. Unplug appliances with clocks when not in use.

EQUIPPING THE GREEN KITCHEN

REUSABLE, LONG-LASTING KITCHENWARE AND ACCESSORIES

It's worth keeping track of your garbage for a few weeks. Watch what you throw away, and ask yourself if each item you are throwing away could be replaced with a reusable substitute. You may see many coffee filters in the trash, for example. Why not buy a gold or cloth reusable coffee filter instead? You may see a lot of Popsicle wrappers. How about investing in good plastic Popsicle molds to make your own? Or plastic sandwich boxes to replace plastic bags for lunches? Not only will you significantly reduce your consumption of resources by using reusable housewares instead of disposables, but you will also save a great deal of money.

Take the simple example of substituting cloth towels for paper towels. At an upstate New York supermarket, recycled paper towels cost $1.59 for 175 sheets. An average family goes through two rolls a week, eight rolls a month, ninety-six rolls a year, at a cost of $152.64. Twelve 100 percent cotton, bird's-eye cotton towels would last about three years, at a cost of $35. For that period you would have spent $457.92 on paper towels, so buying cotton towels would save you $422.92. (Granted, you need to wash the cotton towels, but they don't take up much room in the washing machine and easily can be hung to dry.)

IDEAS FOR REUSABLE INSTEAD OF DISPOSABLE KITCHENWARE

Gold or cloth coffee filters
Cloth towels
Cloth napkins
Durable plastic plates and cups for picnics and birthday parties
Reusable stainless steel utensils for picnics
House water filter, or pour-through water filter pitchers
Travel mug
Reusable baking pans
Cloth bags for shopping—including string bags for produce
Reusable lunch box containers
Reusable plastic Popsicle molds
Plastic containers
Bowl lids (for storage)
Cylinder barbecue starter
Rechargeable household batteries

By using these reusable substitutes, you can cut way back on plastic bags, aluminum foil, paper plates, towels and napkins, plastic wrap, plastic water jugs, paper coffee filters, and more. We are all still faced with packaging waste to throw away, however, as well as worn-out items. But you may be surprised to learn how many items can be reused.

REUSE ITEMS

The list of items you can reuse in your kitchen is lengthy. Glass mustard and mayonnaise jars can be reused to make salad dressings. Old cotton clothing and sheets can be reused for dusting and cleaning rags. (There is nothing like old, soft cotton for a cleaning rag.) Yogurt tubs are great for leftovers. The book *Choose to Reuse,* by Nikki and David Goldbeck, is an invaluable resource for ideas and information about reuse. Not only does the book have suggestions for reusing items you may already have in the home, but it also offers sources of where to have products such as cookware repaired, or where to buy reused equipment and appliances.

HELPFUL EQUIPMENT

There are many choices of kitchen appliances, gadgets, and gizmos available to us. Directing you to which of the many ones you should use lies outside the scope of this book, except to suggest using those that make your cooking experience more convenient and energy efficient. Whether or not to have a crockpot or bread-maker, for example, is your decision, according to how you like to cook. Small appliances are more energy efficient, but not by so much more as to make a big difference (see above). Whether you can buy special steel knives is often a matter of finances. But there are three important appliances that can make a big difference in your ability to produce flavorful, fresh, whole foods in your kitchen: a grinder that grinds grains, spices, and nuts; a steamer for grains and vegetables; and a pressure cooker.

GRINDER FOR GRAINS AND MORE

If you have read chapter 4, "The Green Pantry," you will know that once grains—and many other foods such as spices and nuts—are milled, they lose a great deal of their nutritional value. And the longer between the milling of the grain, grinding of the spices, or chopping of the nuts, the more rancid the natural oils in the foods can get. Grinding your own flours will cost you a fraction of the cost of store-bought. Last but certainly not least, the flavor of freshly ground grains, nuts, and spices is incomparable to that of anything that has been sitting on the shelf for a while.

THE BACK TO BASICS GRINDER

There is one excellent *hand* grinder on the market, the Back to Basics Grinder, that will grind and mill grains, nuts, seeds, and herbs and spices. While refraining from mentioning brand names throughout this book, in this case we are making an exception because this hand grinder is the only one on the market that will mill flour to the finest consistency—the other hand mills only grind coarse flour. It will grind in a range from very fine flour to bulgur to cracked wheat. Electric food mills, discussed below, are excellent and versatile products, but they cost between two and three hundred dollars, which is out of the range of many pocketbooks. The Back to Basics hand grinder retails for sixty dollars. While this is not pocket change, the increased nutritional value of the foods because they are ground on the spot makes it highly worth the cost. The Back to Basics Grinder is also an excellent choice for those who use a moderate amount of flour a day, say two to four cups. You can grind one cup of flour per minute for fine flour, and two cups of flour per minute on the coarse setting. The grinding is easy and there is no "drag," which one often finds with a stone grinder.

The Back to Basics grinding burrs are self-aligning and made of hardened steel alloy. The grinder is adjustable for any desired flour texture and flakes grains very well too. A particularly appealing aspect of this model of hand grinder is that it comfortably grinds nuts, seeds, herbs, and spices also. Because the food isn't milled with stone, which tends to gum up with high-oil-content foods, high-oil flours and even nuts can be ground. While not as good as a food processor for making nut butters, it will quickly grind nuts into small pieces for making breads. Many grind dehydrated vegetables into powders to make vegetable juices. And grinding fresh spices from pods and seeds, to order, results in much more flavorful food. (See "Resources.")

ELECTRIC FLOUR MILLS

Electric flour mills are a deluxe way of grinding grains and beans into flour for baking. Most have many settings, from fine to coarse, and they can usually process six cups of flour at a time, with a nineteen-cup "receiving" pan. The average machine can mill more than one pound of flour a minute. If you bake a lot, this appliance will be a great addition to your life. The King Arthur Flour *Baker's Catalogue* claims that freshly ground grain has a special sweetness compared to grain that has been sitting on the shelf for a while.

Electric flour mills are available from the King Arthur Flour *Baker's Catalogue,* as well as others (see "Resources"). They cost between two and three hundred dollars.

GRAIN STEAMERS/RICE COOKERS/FOOD STEAMERS

Most of the food steamers on the market are rice cookers that can be used for steaming other foods as well. The advantage of using a rice cooker for rice and other grains is that a thermostat will shut the appliance down at the right time for a perfectly cooked product. Many will keep rice warm for many hours—up to twelve hours in some cases. Another reason for using a rice cooker is that it can be the inspiration for cooking a lot of other whole grains as well as rice. You can time grains to be finished and kept warm for a hot breakfast porridge, for example. Or instead of rice for a meal, you can substitute kasha. Turn to chapter 4, "The Green Pantry," for unusual grains to try.

A variety of rice cookers are available. The simplest type of rice cooker will cook the rice and shut the appliance off when it is done. It won't keep the rice warm, but it is safe and effective. The next, more complicated type will cook the rice and then lower the heat to keep the food warm for four hours or so. This can be the least preferable. For one reason, the rice on the bottom of the pan can get thick and glutinous during the warming time. These simpler types of rice cookers cost from between fifty to a hundred dollars. The inner pan is usually aluminum, and they can come with baskets to steam vegetables as well as rice—but almost none recommend you steam a grain and vegetable at the same time.

The next level of rice cooker is electronic, and these will cook rice and keep it warm for up to twelve hours. This cooker circulates the steam throughout so that the rice does not develop a crust on the bottom of the pan. The rice will keep the same consistency as when it was cooked. Some of the electronic rice cookers will also compensate for improper measuring of water and rice. Most of the electronic cookers have a nonstick interior surface and don't have a steaming plate for vegetables, since the plate can scratch the nonstick surface. The rice cookers that keep rice warm for twelve hours are particularly popular in homes where rice and whole grains are a main staple. Electronic units cost from between one and two hundred dollars. Some very top-of-the-line rice cookers are induction heating units, which cook the rice completely evenly. They cost around four hundred dollars.

Make sure the rice cooker you are considering buying can cook brown rice and other grains. You will need to presoak the whole grains and learn the correct water proportions (see chapter 4). It is also prudent to avoid food steamers that have plastic baskets, since the plastic can release fumes when heated. Select a size of rice steamer that cooks about twice as much rice as you usually use, so you can make rice and grains for entertaining. Rice steamers are available in department stores and specialty gourmet stores.

PRESSURE COOKERS

A pressure cooker will cook food very fast and seal in the food's nutrients and flavors. Beans, which generally need to be soaked overnight and boiled for a number of hours, can be cooked in twenty minutes. Rice can be cooked in six minutes. An entire chicken dinner can be done in a flash. Modern-day pressure cookers are safe to use if you follow the directions. If you have an old pressure cooker with a removable "jiggler" valve, you should consider replacing it with a newer version that has a stationary release valve and second safety release. While accidents aren't commonplace with the "jiggler" valve, they do happen, because food can clog the valve, causing too much pressure to build in the pot and the top to blow off.

Until the controversy over the health effects of aluminum leaching from pans is resolved, the prudent choice is a stainless steel pressure cooker. They are available in department stores, kitchen stores, and places that sell kitchen equipment. The cheapest kind available cooks at sixteen pounds pressure and has a valve that pops up and releases. Spend the extra money to get into the price range for a pressure cooker with a second safety release valve. The second safety release usually will open the gasket and release pressure that way. Another safety feature that some pressure cookers have is that they won't pressurize if the top is put on incorrectly (so it won't blow off when under pressure). The middle-line pressure cookers offer both high- and low-steam pressure, so you can do slower cooking at ten pounds pressure, for a pot roast, for example. The top-of-the-line pressure cookers even have a timer that you attach to your shirt or other clothing, to beep you when your food is cooked. Pressure cookers with two safety features range in price from $75 to $200. Electric pressure cookers, which can keep food warm for up to five hours and have an automatic temperature control, cost around $260.

A SPECIAL NOTE ABOUT SPONGES

Many new sponges are impregnated with an antimicrobial agent that kills germs and odors and will last the lifetime of the sponge. This "germ-resistant technology" is incorporated into sponges and sponge scrubbers to such a degree that it is very hard to find a natural cellulose sponge. Antimicrobials are pesticides manufactured for the purpose of killing or inhibiting bacteria and mold. Look for "100 percent natural" on the label of any sponge you buy.

DINNERWARE WITHOUT THE LEAD

Plates and dishes now sold in the United States are subject to federal regulations for the maximum amount of lead they may contain. The state of California has its own stricter regulations for lead. The federal standards require that plates contain no more than 3 ppm lead, and pitchers and other "hollow ware" that hold liquid can contain no more than .5 ppm. The California regulations require that no more than 0.2265 ppm of lead be found in dinnerware, and no more than 0.1 ppm in pitchers or hollow ware.

Because major dinnerware manufacturers sell their dishes in California as well as the rest of the country, if you buy a major brand of dishes you can be quite assured that they meet the stricter California regulations for lead content. To test for lead, the dinnerware is placed in a 4 percent acetic solution for twenty-four hours, and then tested. If you extrapolate from this test you can see that acidic foods pull out the lead. Be particularly cautious about storing juices and wines in containers that could have lead in them. The most serious concern of all is drinking liquid that has been stored in older crystal that was made of lead. In pottery the lead is found in the glazes. When in doubt, ask if the glazes used for the dinnerware you are considering buying are lead free. Be particularly wary of bright red glazes.

POTS AND PANS

Until more is understood about how our bodies handle the small amounts of metals that may leach from cooking pots, one's best choice is to use the most inert cooking utensils available. Porcelain enamel over metals such as steel or iron and glass would be the safest bet from this perspective. As with lead, acidic foods such as spaghetti sauce help leach metals from pans. Avoid high-heat with nonstick coatings, as small amounts of the coating can release fumes into the air. For the same reason, do not use plastics in the microwave.

CLEAN INDOOR AIR

It is very comforting to know that there are no poisons in your kitchen that could hurt your family and to feel that your home is a sanctuary from pollution. There are five main areas of concern about chemical exposure in the kitchen: pesticides, cleaning products, gas stoves, formaldehyde, and contaminated drinking water. Alternatives to pesticides and cleaning products are discussed above, as are water filters.

There are a number of whole house concerns for clean indoor air that affect the kitchen. We highly recommend you test for radon, have all combustion appliances such as oil burners and gas stoves tuned up regularly, install a carbon monoxide detector, determine if your walls are painted with lead paint, reduce the mold in the house, choose carpeting carefully, and even buy or rent a gauss meter to check for high electromagnetic fields. (Real Goods Trading Company sells a gauss meter. See "Resources.") A very good reference book for establishing clean indoor air is *Healthy Homes, Healthy Kids,* by Joyce M. Schoemaker and Charity Y. Vitale. The EPA also provides a lot of public information about indoor air issues (see "Resources").

FORMALDEHYDE

Many of us are subjected to high levels of formaldehyde in our kitchens, from cabinets made of particleboard, pressed wood, and interior grade plywood. Solid wood or metal cabinets are preferable for this reason. If you have particleboard or pressed-wood cabinets, seal in the formaldehyde with sealants made for this purpose. They are available from catalog companies such as N.E.E.D.S. and green stores (see "Resources"). Formaldehyde never completely releases all its fumes from pressed-wood products because it is actually part of the resin that glues the wood chips and sawdust together. Formaldehyde releases fumes at higher levels when heated (a cabinet next to a heater or oven, or direct sunlight, for example) or when exposed to humidity and moisture.

Formaldehyde has been found to cause cancer in animals and industrial workers. It can be a permanent sensitizer, meaning that it can induce sensitivity to lower levels of formaldehyde, and to other chemicals as well. Other symptoms of formaldehyde exposure include sore throat, respiratory tract irritation, nausea, headaches, and asthma.

GAS STOVES

While gas stoves are energy savers, they can cause a significant amount of indoor air pollution, in particular high indoor concentrations of nitrogen dioxide (NO_2). NO_2 can cause increased risk of respiratory tract infection, chronic bronchitis, and eye irritation, and some link increases in childhood colds and flu to even low levels of NO_2. British researchers reported in the medical journal *Lancet* that in a study of 1,159 people, women who cooked with gas stoves were more likely to have asthma than those who cooked on electric. The link was not found in men, but that may be because men tend to cook less than women. In reaction to the report, Dr. Jarvis of St. Thomas Hospital in London estimates that asthma attacks could be reduced by 67 percent if women used electric stoves instead of gas.

If you use a gas stove, make sure that the stove has an exhaust hood and fan to the outside, or at least keep a window open when using the stove. Upgrade to an appliance with electronic ignition instead of a pilot light. Make sure that the flame burns blue and not yellow. If you have questions about how to make your gas stove safer, contact the Gas Appliance Manufacturers Association, Inc. (see "Resources"). Never use your gas stove for heat. Last but not least, on a slightly different note regarding combustion appliances in the kitchen, never cook with charcoal inside your home.

DEALING WITH GARBAGE

Waste is a human concept. In nature nothing is wasted, for everything is part of a continuous cycle. Even the death of a creature provides nutrients that will eventually be reincorporated in the chain of life.

—Denis Hayes, Cofounder of Earth Day

On average, every American throws away more than four pounds of garbage a day. The EPA projects that by the year 2000 the amount will be four and a half pounds. Something has got to change, because there is no safe place for all this garbage to go—landfills are filling up and also leach toxins, and incinerators contaminate surrounding areas with dioxin and more. Those that package our food and other consumer products are mostly responsible for the huge amounts of garbage we throw away, and until they change, it will be hard for us to significantly reduce our garbage. But there is a lot we can do to help the situation, and by careful choices we can at least halve our family's daily contribution to the garbage overload.

David Goldbeck, author of *The Smart Kitchen,* talks of the need to use good kitchen design to reduce barriers to environmental activity. If recycling is made difficult because a convenient system to do so isn't in place, we won't recycle. So the first way to start making less garbage—besides acquiring less packaging in stores—is to set up systems in our homes to make handling our garbage in an environmentally responsible manner more convenient.

Goldbeck offers five principles of recycling system design.

PRINCIPLES OF RECYCLING SYSTEM DESIGN*

1. Design backwards from the local collection system. It is extremely important that the recyclable items not have to be resorted. The key to a good design is to minimize effort on the part of the recycler as this will reduce resistance to recycling. No matter whether the recyclables are to be carried to curbside or recycling center in paper bags, boxes, or cans, the design system must be based on those receptacles.

2. Location factors include site where waste is created, but more important is the distance from the exit used to carry out recyclables as they may be cumbersome and heavy.

3. The recycling area should be made unsuitable to other uses. If the children start putting toys in the containers, or residents their laundry, the system will lose its ability to facilitate recycling. Likewise, avoid holding systems which may get covered up, such as those within benches (except for secondary storage), as this may inhibit their use.

4. Provide a secondary storage area, if possible. This is particularly important where recycling is voluntary and materials may accumulate before being brought to the recycling center.

5. Recycling area should be located in an obvious location and easily used by visitors and future residents.

Reprinted by permission of the author. © David Goldbeck and Ceres Press.

Food Waste

If you collect food scraps for composting you become aware of how much food waste a family can actually go through in a day. Those carrot tops and onion peels can really add up! Some estimate that a full 10 percent of our overall garbage is food scraps, more in vegetarian families. One thing you can do to reduce your food waste is to make vegetable stock with leftover vegetable scraps. The broth will be wonderful and nourishing to add to soups. The other thing you can do with food waste is to compost it.

COMPOSTING

Carrot tops, onion skins, orange peels, and even coffee grounds can be put in an outside pile or bin of some sort, then covered with grass, leaves, and brush to decompose into a rich, dirtlike organic material full of nutrients that makes excellent soil fertilizer and is called compost. You can keep adding layers of fruit and vegetable matter, covering with leaves and grass, making the compost bin or pile your main place to discard food waste.

Basically there are four steps to composting.

1. Choose a composting bin. Available in hardware stores and mail-order catalogs everywhere, composters come in a variety of designs, from a simple wooden slatted box, to large tumbler barrels that can be turned easily. Gardening magazines are full of advertisements for composters and offer 800 numbers for further information. Choose your bin carefully. If you live in the country and have a lot of wild animals, look for an animal-resistant variety of composter. If you use compost for your own garden, and it is a large garden, consider a tumbler barrel composter, which can make usable compost in two weeks.

2. Choose a spot for your compost and a system for getting your compost to the composter. Make sure the compost bin is downwind from your house, and far enough away to keep odors away. You need to be careful not to keep food waste in your kitchen for very long because molds grow very

quickly on it, which can be a serious issue for anyone with mold allergies. Keep a colander in your sink, or a bucket with a tightly covered top, to store food waste for no more than a day or two. Make sure not to put animal products in the compost.

3. The commonly used composting mixture is four parts green compost to two parts brown compost. Green compost consists of food scraps, weeds, grass cuttings, and green trimmings and is high in nitrogen. Brown compost consists of dead leaves, branches, brush, straw, and wood shavings and is high in carbon. Every time you place green compost in the pile, add half as much brown compost on top.

4. Mix regularly. If you turn the pile once or twice a week the compost will decompose faster and not smell as much.

Once you have compost you can use it to fertilize gardens, trees, and plants. If you don't use it yourself, there is many a gardener who would be happy to have it. Some farmers may take fresh kitchen scraps. If you live in the city, ask farmers selling at your farmers' market.

ESPECIALLY FOR THOSE IN THE CITY: WORM COMPOSTING

If you live in a city you can compost your garbage in a worm composting bin—no fuss, no mess.

Deborah Highly's husband gave her a worm bin for Christmas. While not high on the Christmas list of most, a worm bin was what Deborah wanted, even though she lived in the country, because she thought that an outdoor compost pile might attract animals. She describes worm composting as a very simple process with a few steps.

1. Get a bin with air holes on the side. They are available from Seventh Generation and Real Goods Trading Company catalogs. (See "Resources.") You get the worms separately. You cover the bottom of the bin with newspaper and water, in a ratio of three times more newspaper than water. (One gallon of water equals eight pounds.) If there is too little water the worms will die.

2. You can get your worms from local gardening shops or fishing supply stores. Buy red worms. If you buy worms from bait stores they will be more expensive and they will be too big; little worms are more adaptive. You can also order the worms from mail-order sources. They can survive for two weeks without food. The basic formula is that two pounds of worms will handle the food waste of a family of four to six, while one pound of worms will handle the waste from a family of two.
3. Measure your garbage. Two pounds of worms will eat one pound of garbage a day. If you overfeed the worms the bin will begin to smell.
4. Harvest the bin every two to three months. To harvest, you separate the worms from the dirt (which is their excrement—vermicompost—and can be used as fertilizer) by making small piles on newspaper and gently shaking the piles to separate the worms.

Recycling and Waste*

Don't put hazardous waste in the garbage because it can leach into landfills and ultimately into the water supply, or be incinerated, releasing toxins into the air. Hazardous waste includes auto maintenance (motor oil, transmission fluid and additives, engine lubricants, antifreeze, windshield wiper solution, lead-acid batteries, engine cleaners and solvents, gas treatments, gas line freeze-up products, and car waxes. Outside use products (fertilizers, pesticides, pool chemicals, self-lighting charcoal, charcoal lighter fluid, butane lighters; hobby and repair products; paintbrush cleaner, sprays and aerosols, lacquers and thinners, alcohol (not for human consumption), cresol, naphtha, mineral spirits, turpentine, wood preservatives, glues and adhesives, photographic chemicals. Cleaning products; furniture polishes and stains, floor waxes, car waxes, spray dust cleaners, drain cleaners, toilet bowl cleaners, oven cleaners, spot and stain removers (petroleum based), all aerosols, shoe polish.

*Adapted from the Vermont Agency of Natural Resources.

Packaging Made of Plastic, Paper, Glass, and Aluminum

Every town and city in the country has a different capacity for recycling packaging waste. All discussion here about recycling is meaningless unless it applies specifically to your community. Call your town's or city's recycling center. Most have brochures to offer you and clear guidelines for you to follow.

The less packaging waste you will have for the landfill or incinerator, the better. See chapter 3 for suggestions on how to reduce the amount and types of packaging you bring home from the store.

PLASTIC

It is obvious to anybody who has felt the dissimilarity between a plastic lunchbox and a polystyrene coffee cup that there are many different kinds of plastics. It might not be so obvious that the various plastics are actually made up of different ingredients. All plastics have in common a base of different nonrenewable crude oil compounds, but each kind of plastic is formed from different crude-oil-based compounds and may be bound together with different chemical additives and resins. These variations make some plastics recyclable and others not, and some more damaging to health and the environment than others.

Recognizing the different kinds of plastic is easy with the help of the three arrows that form a triangular shape with a number in the center found on the bottom of plastic containers. Some letters appear below the three arrows that form the triangular shape, and these represent the kind of resin used to make the plastic. By understanding the numbers (see below), you can begin to make educated choices about plastics—what kinds of plastic packaging can be recycled, what kinds you can never recycle, and what kinds you should avoid whenever possible because they are so damaging to the environment.

Every plastic package you buy that contains food of any kind (except for polystyrene egg cartons, berry baskets, and soda bottles) is made completely out of virgin resources. Because plastic is recycled at a temperature too low to ensure complete sterilization of the containers, it is never recycled for use with food.

According to the EPA, in 1994 only 7.6 percent of plastic garbage was recycled. To reduce our own contributions to incinerators and already overburdened landfills, we need to limit how much food we buy that is packaged in plastic. Try hard to buy food packaged only in plastic that is recyclable (and then recycle it!), or at least reusable.

Plastic Identification Symbols

Symbol No. 1

PETE, PET (polyethylene terephthalate). PET is commonly recycled, but there is a lot of pollution generated in its manufacture. You can further identify PET soda bottles because they do not have side seams.

Common Packaging: Soda bottles (PET is the only plastic that can contain carbonated drinks), boil-in-a-bag foods, some spring-water, juices, liquid cleaning products, and cosmetics.

Recycled Uses: A wide range of textiles and fibers such as sleeping bags, carpet fibers, pillows, twine, fiberfill jackets, fiberfill insulation, and polyester. Also recycled into engineering plastics, some vegetable oil containers, plastic liquor bottles, paintbrushes, scouring pads, containers, biodegradable plastic bags, and six-pack carriers.

Note: Make sure to remove bottle caps and plastic bottle collars before recycling. They are made of plastic no. 5 and are not currently recycled.

Symbol No. 2

HDPE (high-density polyethylene). HDPE is commonly recycled. One of the plastics with the least environmental impact, it is commonly used to package consumer products.

Common Packaging: Plastic bottles such as milk, water, and juice jugs; liquid detergents, bleach, and fabric softeners; shampoos; pharmaceutical products; butter and other dairy containers; some plastic grocery bags; automotive products such as windshield wiper fluid and motor oil.

Recycled Uses: Trash bins, traffic cones, plastic lumber, base cups for soft drink containers, crates, flowerpots, and much more.

Note: Make sure to remove bottle caps and plastic bottle collars before recycling. They are made of plastic no. 5 and are not currently recycled.

Symbol No. 3

V/PVC (vinyl/polyvinyl chloride). Avoid this plastic. Some estimates are that about 34 percent of global chlorine production is used to make PVC. PVC is a significant source of dioxin in the environment; dioxin can be produced during its manufacture and incineration. Because it is the least recyclable of all plastics, PVC often ends up in incinerators, where it releases not only dioxin but also carcinogens such as PCBs.

Common Packaging: Bottles of floor wax, shampoos, vegetable oils, salad dressing, mouthwashes, mineral water, and lunch meat wrap.

Recycled Uses: Construction pipes, such as for drainage and sewer; vinyl floor tiles; house siding; truck-bed liners.

Note: Never recycle no. 3 with other plastics.

Symbol No. 4

LDPE (low-density polyethylene). Not currently recycled.

Common Packaging: Plastic squeeze bottles, cosmetics, plastic sandwich bags, grocery bags, and most shrink-wrap packaging.

Recycled Uses: None.

Note: LDPE doesn't make a crinkly sound when crushed.

Symbol No. 5

PP (polypropylene). Not currently recycled. Less polluting than most plastic to manufacture.

Common Packaging: Some dairy products such as yogurt and cottage cheese; plastic bottles; foods that are packaged hot, such as syrups; caps on jars and bottles; syrup bottles.

Recycled Uses: None.

Symbol No. 6

PS (polystyrene). Some versions of polystyrene are known as Styrofoam. Styrene, from which polystyrene is made, is very toxic and a possible carcinogen. Manufacture of polystyrene causes large amounts of hazardous waste.

Common Packaging: Pharmaceutical ingredients such as tablets and creams; cups and saucers; foam hot drink cups; foam packing material such as packing peanuts; meat, fish, and poultry trays; egg cartons; some fast-food restaurant take-out packaging; molded foam for packing electronic equipment such as computers; clear plastic salad bar take-out containers.

Recycled Uses: Plastic lumber.

Reuse Options: There are many places around the country that take back polystyrene packing peanuts. For information, call the association of foam packaging recyclers at 800-944-9449.

Symbol No. 7

Other (primarily multilayered plastics). It is very hard to find places to recycle multilayered plastics, so it usually ends up in incinerators or landfills.

Common Packaging: Aseptic packaging.

Recycled Uses: Plastic lumber, paper.

Basic Guidelines for Choosing, Reusing, Refilling, or Recycling Plastic Food Packaging

1. Avoid food packaged in plastic whenever possible.
2. Contact your local government for information about what plastics are recyclable in your community, and how to recycle those items. Stick as much as you can to buying only plastic that is recyclable in your community.
3. Of all the plastics, the best choice is no. 2, HDPE, because it is one of the easiest plastics to recycle and does not pollute as much during either its manufacture or incineration as other plastics. Plastic no. 1 is also easy to recycle but causes more pollution in its manufacture.
4. Plastics nos. 3 through 7 do not have much of a market for recycling and are hard to recycle in most communities.
5. Try to reuse plastics whenever possible by purchasing refillable products, a service provided in many health food stores.
6. When you recycle be scrupulous not to mix plastics, as doing so contaminates the recycling process, since many plastic resins cannot be mixed.

7. A rule of thumb many recycling centers suggest for determining if a plastic is recyclable is the "stomp test." "Stomp" on the container, and if it cracks or breaks into pieces, it cannot be recycled.

8. If you plan to reuse plastic, make sure it is thoroughly sterilized before doing so. When in doubt, throw it out.

9. So-called biodegradable plastics—those marketed to biodegrade naturally within a few years (most plastics take centuries to biodegrade)—require light to biodegrade, therefore they will not biodegrade buried in landfills.

PAPER

According to the EPA, in 1994, 45.2 percent of paper and paperboard trash was recycled. To recycle paper packaging, first call your recycling center to determine how they categorize and separate the paper types. Many recycling centers will accept "mixed paper." This category is great for recycling cereal boxes, nonaluminum wrapping paper, toilet roll tubes, and more. Most recycling centers also have a special category for brown paper bags and cartons.

Recycling magazines printed on glossy paper is difficult to do throughout the country.

ALUMINUM AND STEEL PACKAGING

According to the EPA, in 1994, 55 percent of aluminum trash was recycled. There probably isn't a recycling center in the country that won't accept cans. Wash the cans thoroughly, take off the paper label (to recycle in the "mixed paper" container), use a can opener to take off the top and bottom of the can, and flatten the can. "Can crushers" are available in green stores and catalogs. (Some recycling centers and supermarkets with machines that accept cans for recycling require that cans not be crushed.) Aluminum foil can be recycled. Reynolds Metals has established drop-off centers for aluminum foil around the country. Look in the yellow pages under "Recycling, aluminum." The vast majority of beer and soft drink cans are aluminum.

In 1994, 51 percent of steel packaging—primarily canned foods—was recycled, according to the EPA.

GLASS

According to the EPA, in 1994, 25.8 percent of the glass trash in the United States was recycled. Because glass is 100 percent recyclable, each pound of glass you recycle can be transformed into one pound of "new" glass, and it can continue to be recycled forever. To recycle glass, wash it thoroughly, take off the paper label if possible (to recycle in the "mixed paper" container), and recycle without tops.

LARGE APPLIANCES

Call your electric company to find out where to recycle refrigerators. You want to find a place that will recycle both freon and CFCs. Nearly 85 percent of CFCs in refrigerators are contained in their insulating foam, so make sure the company that takes your fridge has the appropriate equipment.

Appendix
Nutritional Data

Beans (1 cup cooked)

	Protein/Grams	Fat/Grams	Carbohydrates/Grams	Calories	Fiber/Grams	Calcium	Iron	Magnesium	Phosphorus	Potassium	Sodium	Zinc	Copper	Manganese	Vitamin A/I.U.	Ascorbic Acid	Thiamin	Riboflavin	Niacin	Pantothenic Acid	Vitamin B6	Folacin/Micrograms	Vitamin B12/Micrograms
Adzuki beans	17	0.2	57	294	N/A	64	7	120	386	1223	18	4	0.7	1	14	0	0.3	0.1	2	1	0.2	278	0
Black beans	15	0.9	41	227	15	46	4	120	241	610	2	2	0.4	0.8	N/A	0	0.4	0.1	0.9	0.4	0.1	256	0
Chickpeas	14	4	45	269	N/A	80	5	79	275	477	11	2	0.6	2	44	2	0.2	0.1	0.9	0.5	0.2	282	0
Great Northern beans	15	0.8	37	203	12	120	4	88	292	672	3	1	0.4	0.9	2	2	0.3	0.1	1	0.5	0.2	181	0
Kidney beans	15	0.9	40	225	11	49	5	80	251	713	3	2	0.4	0.8	0	2	0.3	0.1	1	0.4	0.2	229	0
Lentils	18	0.7	40	230	16	38	6	71	356	730	4	2	0.5	1	16	3	0.3	0.1	2	1	0.3	358	0
Lima beans	15	0.7	39	216	13	32	4	81	208	955	4	2	0.4	1	0	0	0.3	0.1	0.8	0.8	0.3	156	0

Food	Vitamin B12/Micrograms	Folacin/Micrograms	Vitamin B6	Pantothenic Acid	Niacin	Riboflavin	Thiamin	Ascorbic Acid	Vitamin A/I.U.	Manganese	Copper	Zinc	Sodium	Potassium	Phosphorus	Magnesium	Iron	Calcium	Fiber/Grams	Calories	Carbohydrates/Grams	Fat/Grams	Protein/Grams
Mung beans, raw	0	1293	0.8	4	5	0.5	1	10	2	236	2	5	31	2579	760	391	14	273	34	718	130	2	49
Mung beans, cooked	0	321	0.1	0.8	1	0.1	0.3	2	48	0.6	0.3	2	4	537	200	97	3	54	15	212	39	0.8	14
Navy beans	0	254	0.3	0.5	1	0.1	0.4	1	4	1	0.5	2	2	670	286	107	4	127	N/A	258	48	1	16
Pinto beans	0	294	0.2	0.5	0.7	0.1	0.3	4	3	0.9	0.4	2	3	800	273	94	4	82	15	234	44	0.9	14
Soybeans	0	92	0.4	0.3	0.7	0.5	0.2	3	15	1	0.7	2	2	886	421	148	9	175	10	297	17	15	29
Split peas	0	127	0.09	1	2	0.1	0.4	0.8	14	0.8	0.3	2	4	709	194	70	2	27	16	231	41	0.7	16

Flours (1 cup)

Food	Vitamin B12/Micrograms	Folacin/Micrograms	Vitamin B6	Pantothenic Acid	Niacin	Riboflavin	Thiamin	Ascorbic Acid	Vitamin A/I.U.	Manganese	Copper	Zinc	Sodium	Potassium	Phosphorus	Magnesium	Iron	Calcium	Fiber/Grams	Calories	Carbohydrates/Grams	Fat/Grams	Protein/Grams
Buckwheat flour	0	65	0.7	0.5	7	0.2	0.5	0	0	2	0.6	4	13	692	404	301	5	49	12	402	85	4	15
Cornmeal	0	31	0.4	0.5	4	0.2	0.5	0	572	0.6	0.2	2	43	350	294	155	4	7	9	442	94	4	10
Brown rice flour	0	25	1	2	10	0.1	0.7	0	0	6	0.3	4	12	457	532	177	3	17	7	574	120	4	11
Dark rye flour	0	77	0.5	2	5	0.3	0.4	0	0	8	1	7	1	934	809	317	8	72	29	415	88	3	18
Triticale flour	0	96	0.5	3	4	0.2	0.5	0	0	5	0.7	3	3	606	417	199	3	45	19	439	95	2	17
Whole wheat flour	0	53	0.4	1	7	0.2	0.5	0	0	4	0.5	3	6	486	415	166	5	44	14	407	87	2	16

Grains (1cup)

Grains (1cup)	Protein/Grams	Fat/Grams	Carbohydrates/Grams	Calories	Fiber/Grams	Calcium	Iron	Magnesium	Phosphorus	Potassium	Sodium	Zinc	Copper	Manganese	Vitamin A/I.U.	Ascorbic Acid	Thiamin	Riboflavin	Niacin	Pantothenic Acid	Vitamin B6	Folacin/Micrograms	Vitamin B12/Micrograms
Amaranth	28	13	129	729	30	298	14	518	887	714	41	6	1	4	0	8	0.2	0.4	2	2	0.4	95	0
Barley, dry	23	4	134	690	32	61	7	245	486	832	22	5	0.9	3	40	0	1	0.5	7	0.5	0.6	35	0
Brown rice, long	5	2	45	216	3	19	0.8	84	162	84	10	1	0.2	1.7	0	0	0.2	0.05	3	0.5	0.3	8	0
Barley, pearled, cooked	3	0.7	44	193	6	17	2	34	85	146	5	1	0.1	0.4	11	0	0.1	0.1	3	0.2	0.2	25	0
Bulgur, cooked	5	0.4	34	151	8	18	2	58	73	124	9	1	0.1	1	0	0	0.1	0.05	2	6	0.1	33	0
Millet	8	2	57	286	3	7	1	105	240	149	5	2	0.4	0.6	0	0	0.2	0.2	3	0.4	0.3	46	0
Oats	26	11	103	606	N/A	84	7	276	816	669	3	6	1	7	0	0	1	0.2	1	2	0.2	87	0
Quinoa	22	10	117	636	10	102	16	357	697	1258	36	6	1	4	0	0	0.3	0.7	5	2	0.4	83	0
Rye, dry	25	4	118	566	25	56	4	204	632	446	10	6	0.7	4	0	0	0.5	0.4	7	2	0.5	101	0
Sorghum	22	6	143	651	N/A	54	8	N/A	551	672	11	N/A	N/A	N/A	0	0	0.4	0.3	5	N/A	N/A	N/A	0
Tapioca, dry	0.3	0.03	135	518	-	30	2	1	11	17	1	0.2	0.03	0.1	0	0	0.006	0	0	0.2	0	6	0
Triticale	25	4	138	645	N/A	71	5	250	687	637	10	6	0.9	6	0	0	0.8	0.2	3	2	0.3	140	0

	Protein/Grams	Fat/Grams	Carbohydrates/Grams	Calories	Fiber/Grams	Calcium	Iron	Magnesium	Phosphorus	Potassium	Sodium	Zinc	Copper	Manganese	Vitamin A/I.U.	Ascorbic Acid	Thiamin	Riboflavin	Niacin	Pantothenic Acid	Vitamin B₆	Folacin/Micrograms	Vitamin B₁₂/Micrograms
Wheat, durum	26	5	136	651	N/A	65	7	276	975	827	4	8	1	6	0	0	0.8	0.2	13	2	0.8	83	0
Wheat, red spring	30	4	131	632	24	48	7	238	637	653	4	5	0.8	8	0	0	1	0.2	11	2	0.6	82	0
Wild rice, cooked	6	0.5	35	166	3	5	1	52	134	165	5	2	0.2	0.5	0	0	0.08	0.1	2	0.2	0.2	43	0
Soy products																							
Soy milk (1 cup)	7	4	4	79	3	10	1	46	118	338	29	0.5	0.3	0.4	77	0	0.4	0.2	0.3	0.1	0.1	4	0
Tahini (1 tablespoon)	2	8	3	89	1	64	1	14	110	62	17	0.7	0.2	0.2	10	0	0.2	0.07	0.8	0.1	0.02	15	0
Tamari (1 tablespoon)	2	0.01	1	11	0.1	3	0.4	7	23	38	1005	0.07	0.02	0.09	0	0	0.01	0.02	0.7	0.06	0.03	3	0
Tempeh (¼ pound)	31	13	28	330	N/A	15	4	116	342	609	10	3	1	2	0	0	0.2	0.1	8	0.6	0.5	86	1
Tofu, raw, firm (½ pound)	20	11	5	183	3	258	13	118	298	18	2	2	0.5	1	209	0.2	0.2	0.1	0.5	0.2	0.1	37	0

Nuts and Seeds (1 cup)

	Protein/Grams	Fat/Grams	Carbohydrates/Grams	Calories	Fiber/Grams	Calcium	Iron	Magnesium	Phosphorus	Potassium	Sodium	Zinc	Copper	Manganese	Vitamin A/I.U.	Ascorbic Acid	Thiamin	Riboflavin	Niacin	Pantothenic Acid	Vitamin B6	Folacin/Micrograms	Vitamin B12/Micrograms
Almonds	28	74	29	836	15	378	5	420	738	1039	16	4	1	3	0	0.8	0.3	1	5	0.7	0.2	83	0
Almond butter (1 tablespoon)	2	9	3	101	0.6	43	0.6	48	84	121	2	0.5	0.1	0.4	0	0.1	0.02	0.09	0.5	0.04	0.01	10	0
Brazil nuts	20	93	18	918	8	246	5	315	840	840	3	6	2	1	0	1	1	0.2	2	0.3	0.3	5	0
Butternuts	25	57	12	612	5	53	4	237	446	421	1	3	0.4	6	124	3	0.4	0.1	1	0.6	0.5	66	0
Cashews, dry roasted	21	63	45	786	4	62	8	356	671	774	22	8	3	1	0	0	0.3	0.3	2	1	0.3	0.9	0
Chestnuts, raw	1	1	44	196	N/A	19	0.9	30	38	484	2	0.5	0.4	0.3	26	40	0.1	0	1	0.5	0.3	58	0
Filberts	15	72	17	779	7	216	4	328	359	512	3	3	2	2	77	1	0.6	0.1	1	1	0.7	82	0
Macadamia nuts	11	99	1	1007	12	94	3	3	155	182	493	7	2	0.4	0.8	0	0	0.5	0.1	3	0.6	0.3	0

	Protein/Grams	Fat/Grams	Carbohydrates/Grams	Calories	Fiber/Grams	Calcium	Iron	Magnesium	Phosphorus	Potassium	Sodium	Zinc	Copper	Manganese	Vitamin A I.U.	Ascorbic Acid	Thiamin	Riboflavin	Niacin	Pantothenic Acid	Vitamin B₆	Folacin/Micrograms	Vitamin B₁₂/Micrograms
Peanuts	38	72	23	828	12	134	7	245	549	1029	26	5	2	3	0	0	0.9	0.2	17	3	0.5	350	0
Peanut butter, with salt (1 tablespoon)	4	8	3	94	0.9	5	0.3	25	52	115	76	0.4	0.08	.2	0	0	22	0.01	2	0.1	0.06	12	0
Pecans	8	73	20	720	8	39	2	138	314	423	1	6	1	5	138	2	0.9	0.1	1	2	0.2	42	0
Pine nuts	54	115	32	1169	10	59	21	529	1153	1359	9	10	2	10	66	4.3	2	0.4	8	0.4	0.2	130	0
Pistachios	26	62	32	738	14	173	9	202	644	1400	8	2	1	0.4	298	9	1	0.2	1	1	0.3	74	0
Pumpkin seeds	12	12	34	285	N/A	35	2	168	59	588	11	7	0.4	0.3	40	0.2	0.02	0.03	0.2	0.03	0.02	6	0
Sesame seeds	25	34	34	825	17	1404	21	505	906	674	16	11	6	3	13	0	1	0.3	6	0.07	1	139	0
Sunflower seeds	33	71	27	821	15	167	10	510	1015	992	4	7	2	3	72	2	3	0.4	6	10	1	327	0
Walnuts, black	30	71	15	759	6	72	4	252	580	655	1	4	1	5	370	4	0.3	1	0.9	0.8	0.7	82	0
Walnuts, English	17	74	22	770	6	113	3	203	380	602	12	3	2	3	149	4	0.5	0.2	1	0.7	0.7	79	0

Resources

Chapter 1

PUBLICATIONS

Dietary Guidelines for Americans, Third Edition, 1990, the U.S. Department of Agriculture and the U.S. Department of Health and Human Services (Home and Garden Bulletin No. 232).

"Dietary Guidelines for Sustainability," Joan Dye Gussow and Katherine L. Clancy, *Journal of Nutrition Education* 18, no. 1 (1986).

Eight Steps to the New Green Diet, Wendy Gordon, Mothers & Others for a Livable Planet, New York, 1995.

ORGANIZATIONS

American Farmland Trust, 1920 N Street, NW, Suite 400, Washington, DC 20036; 202-659-5170.

Campaign for Sustainable Agriculture, 12 N. Church Street, Goshen, NY 10924; 914-294-0633.

Healthy Harvest Society, 1424 16th Street, NW, Suite 105, Washington, DC 20036; 202-462-8800.

International Alliance for Sustainable Agriculture, Newman Center, University of Minnesota, 1701 University Avenue SE, Minneapolis, MN 55414; 612-331-1099.

The Land Stewardship Project, 14758 Ostlund Trail North, Marine on St. Croix, MN 55047; 612-433-2770.

Chapter 2

PUBLICATIONS

Becoming Vegetarian, Vesanto Melina, Brenda Davis, Victoria Harrison, Book Publishing Company, Summertown, TN, 1995.

The Book of Apples, Trafalgar Square, Box 257, North Pomfret, VT 05053.

The Book of Whole Meals, Annemarie Colbin, Ballantine Books, New York, 1993.

Chicken Little, Tomato Sauce and Agriculture, Joan Dye Gussow, Bootstrap Press, New York, 1991.

"Dietary Guidelines for Sustainability," Joan Dye Gussow and Katherine L. Clancy, *Journal of Nutrition Education* 18, no. 1 (1986).

Eight Steps to the New Green Diet, Wendy Gordon, Mothers & Others for a Livable Planet, New York, 1995.

"Fat Is Not Just to Keep Your Pants Up: Essential Oil Deficiency," Sidney Baker, *Green Alternatives* 2, no. 3 (1992): pp. 35, 37, 39.

Fats that Heal, Fats that Kill, Udo Erasmus, Alive Books, Durnaby, BC, 1986, 1993.

Food Additives, Ruth Winter, Crown Publishers, New York, 1989.

Healing with Whole Foods: Oriental Traditions and Modern Nutrition, Paul Pitchford, North Atlantic Books, Berkeley, CA, 1993.

The Heirloom Gardener, Carolyn Jabs, Sierra Club Books, San Francisco, 1984.

Our Stolen Future, Theo Colborn, Dianne Damnoski, and John Peterson Myers, Dutton, New York, 1996.

Rain Forest in Your Kitchen, Martin Teitel, Island Press, Washington, DC, 1992.

Safe Food, Michael F. Jacobson, Lisa Y. Lefferts, and Anne Witte Garland, Living Planet Press, Los Angeles, 1991.

Seeds of Change, Kenny Ausubel, Harper San Francisco, San Francisco, 1994.

The Way We Grow, Anne Witte Garland with Mothers & Others for a Livable Planet, Berkley Books, New York, 1993.

ORGANIZATIONS

Classical Fruits, 8831 AL Highway 157, Moulton, AL 35650.

The Seed Savers Exchange, Rte. 3, Box 239, Decorah, IA 52101; 319-382-5990.

Seeds of Change, 1364 Rufina Circle No. 5, Santa Fe, NM 87501; 505-438-8080.

Note: If the seed is a patented hybrid, the word *hybrid* is usually included in the name of the seed.

Chapter 3

PUBLICATIONS

Basic Formula to Create Community Supported Agriculture, Robyn Van En (updated regularly), Indian Line Farm, and *Not Just about Vegetables* video, by Indian Line Farm, Great Barrington, MA.

Eat the Weeds, Ben Charles Harris, Keats Publishing, New Canaan, CT, 1969.

Exploring Nature's Uncultivated Garden, Deborah Lee, Havelin Communications, Inc., Asheville, NC, 1989.

Farms of Tomorrow, Community Supported Farms, Farm Supported Communities, Trauger M. Groh and Steven S. H. McFadden, Bio-dynamic Farming and Gardening Association, Inc., Kimberton, PA, 1990.

The Harvest Times, edited by Melody Newcombe; newsletter for CSA growers. P.O. Box 27, Mt. Tremper, NY 12457; 800-516-7797.

Identifying and Harvesting Edible and Medicinal Plants in Wild (and Not So Wild) Places, "Wildman" Steve Brill with Evelyn Dean, Hearst Books, New York, 1994.

The New Organic Grower's Four-Season Harvest, Eliot Coleman, Chelsea Green Publishing Company, Post Mills, VT, 1992.

The Peterson Guide to Edible Plants, Lee Peterson, Houghton Mifflin, Boston, 1982.

Rodale's Encyclopedia of Organic Gardening, Fern Marshall Bradley and Barbara W. Ellis, eds., Rodale Press, Emmaus, PA, 1992.

Wild Roots: A Forager's Guide to the Edible and Medicinal Roots, Tubers, Corms, and Rhizomes of North America, Doug Elliott, Healing Arts Press, Rochester, VT, 1995.

ORGANIZATIONS

The American Farmland Trust, 1920 N Street, NW, Washington, DC 20036; 202-659-5170.

Appropriate Technology Transfer for Rural Areas (ATTRA), P.O. Box 3657, Fayettesville, AR 72702; 800-346-9140; established by the U.S. Department of Agriculture Extension Service.

Bio-dynamic Farming and Gardening Association in Kimberton, PA; 610-935-7797; 800-516-7797.

Co-op Directory Services, 919 21st Avenue S., Minneapolis, MN 55404; 612-332-0417. For information, send an SASE.

Indian Line Farm, RR 3, Box 85, Great Barrington, MA 01230; 413-528-4374.

Deborah Lee, Health Unlimited, 130 Belle Dame, Lafayette, LA 70506; 318-988-5090. Workshops in medicinals.

National Cooperative Business Association, 1401 New York Avenue, NW, Suite 1000, Washington, DC 20005; 202-638-6222.

United States Department of Agriculture, P.O. Box 96456, Washington, DC 20090-6456; 202-720-8317.

ORGANIC FOOD CATALOGS

Gold Mine Natural Food Company, 1947 30th Street, San Diego, CA 92102; 800-475-FOOD.

Jaffe Brothers, P.O. Box 636, Valley Center, CA 92082-0636; 619-749-1133.

Walnut Acres, Penns Creek, PA 17862; 800-433-3998.

Chapter 4

PUBLICATIONS

Baking Bread, Old and New Traditions, Beth Hensperger, Chronicle Books, San Francisco, 1992.

The Book of Food, Frances Bissell, Henry Holt and Company, New York, 1994.

Boutique Bean Pot, Kathleen Mayes and Sandra Gottfried, Woodbridge Press, Santa Barbara, CA, 1992.

Bread Alone, Daniel Leader and Judith Blahnik, William Morrow and Company, Inc., New York, 1993.

The Brilliant Bean, Sally and Martin Stone, Bantam Books, New York, 1988.

Fats that Heal, Fats that Kill, Udo Erasmus, Alive Books, Durnaby, BC, 1986, 1993.

Grains for Better Health, Maureen B. Keane and Daniella Chace, Prima Publishing, Rocklin, CA, 1994.

Good Food: The Complete Guide to Eating Well, Margaret M. Wittenberg, Crossing Press, 1995.

Gourmet Grains, Maindishes Made of Nature, Candia Lea Cole, Woodbridge Press, Santa Barbara, CA 1991.

Rodale's Illustrated Encyclopedia of Herbs, Claire Kowalchik and William H. Hylton, eds., Rodale Press, Emmaus, PA, 1987.

SOURCES OF HERBS FOR TEA

Blessed Herbs, 109 Barre Plains Road, Oaklam, MA 01068; 800-489-4372.

Companion Plants, 7247 North Coolville Rodige Road, Athens, OH 45701; 614-592-4643.

Granum, Inc., 2901 NE Blakely, Seattle, WA 98105-3120; 206-525-0051.

Herbs, Etc., 1345 Cerrillos Road, Santa Fe, NM 87501; 505-982-1265.

Chapter 5

PUBLICATIONS

The Busy Person's Guide to Preserving Food, Janet Bachand Chadwick, Garden Way Publishers, Charlotte, VT, 1982.

The Complete Book of Home Freezing, Hazel Meyer, Lippincott, Philadelphia, 1953.

The Complete Book of Home Preserving, Ann Seranne, Doubleday, New York, 1955.

Fresh Food, Dirt Cheap, the editors of *Organic Gardening,* Rodale Press, Emmaus, PA, 1981.

The Herbal Tea Garden: Planning, Planting, Harvesting and Brewing, Marieta Marshall Marcin, A Garden Way Publishing Book, Storey Communications, Pownal, VT, 1993.

Home Food Systems, Roger B. Yepsen Jr., ed., Rodale Press, Emmaus, PA, 1981.

How to Dry Fruits and Vegetables at Home, food editors of *Farm Journal,* Countryside Press, Philadelphia, PA, 1975.

Putting Food By, Janet Greene, Ruth Hertzberg, and Beatrice Vaughan, Penguin, New York, 1991.

Stocking Up, Carol Hupping Stoner, ed., Rodale Press, Emmaus, PA, 1977.

CATALOG COMPANIES

McMasters Catalog, P.O. Box 440, New Brunswick, NJ 08903; 908-329-3200 (wire screen).

Chapter 6

PUBLICATIONS

Buy Smart, Buy Safe: A Consumer's Guide to Less-Toxic Products, Philip Dickey, Washington Toxics Coalition (4516 University Way NE, Seattle, WA 98105; 206-632-1545).

Choose to Reuse: An Encyclopedia of Services, Products, Programs and Charitable Organizations, David and Nikki Goldbeck, Ceres Press, Woodstock, NY, 1995.

Clean & Green: The Complete Guide to Nontoxic and Environmentally Safe Housekeeping, Annie Berthold-Bond, Ceres Press, Woodstock, NY, 1990.

Common Sense Pest Control: Least-Toxic Solutions for Your Home, Garden, Pets and Community, William Olkowski, Sheila Daar, and Helga Olkowski, Taunton Press, Newtown, CT, 1991.

Consumer Guide to Home Energy Savings, Alex Wilson and John Morril, American Council for an Energy-Efficient Economy, 1995 (1001 Connecticut Avenue, NW, Suite 801, Washington, DC 20036). Updated regularly.

The Earth and You, Eating for Two, April Moore, Potomac Valley Press, Washington, DC, 1993.

Germany, Garbage and the Green Dot, Betty Fishbein, a publication of INFORM, Inc. (120 Wall Street, New York, NY 10005-4001; 212-361-2400).

Healthy Homes, Healthy Kids, Joyce M. Schoemaker and Charity Y. Vitale, Island Press, Washington, DC, 1991.

Homemade Money, Richard Heede and the staff of Rocky Mountain Institute, Brick House Publishing Company, Amherst, NH, 1995.

The Smart Kitchen: How to Design a Comfortable, Safe, Energy-Efficient, and Environment-Friendly Workspace, David Goldbeck, Ceres Press, Woodstock, NY, 1989.

Turn off the Tap Before It's Too Late, Randall D. Schultz, EccoTime, Albuquerque, NM, 1991.

ORGANIZATIONS

Gas Appliance Manufacturers Association, Inc., 1901 North Moore Street, Suite 1100, Arlington, VA 22209.

Guide to technologies for using a home's gray water system: Metamorphic Press, P.O. Box 1841, Santa Rosa, CA 95402; 707-874-2606.

Plans for making your own solar cooker: Kerr Enterprises, P.O. Box 27417, Tempe, AZ 85285; 602-968-3068.

Public Information Center (PM–211B), U.S. Environmental Protection Agency, 401 M Street, SW, Washington, DC 20460.

Rachel Carson Council, 8940 Jones Mill Road, Chevy Chase, MD 20815; 301-652-1877.

Solar Box Cookers International, 1724 11th Street, Sacramento, CA 95814; 916-444-6616.

CATALOG COMPANIES

Back to Basics Products, Inc., 11660 South State Street, Draper, UT 84020; 800-688-1989 (grain grinders and pressure canners).

The Baker's Catalogue, P.O. Box 876, Norwich, VT 05055-0876.

Lehman's Non-electric Catalog, Box 41, Dept. 2-FBN, Kidron, OH 44636.

N.E.E.D.S., 527 Charles Avenue, Syracuse, NY 13209; 800-711-1123.

Nutriflex, P.O. Box 65409, Salt Lake City, UT 84165-0409; 800-888-8587.

Real Goods Trading Company, 555 Leslie Street, Ukiah, CA 95482-5576; 800-762-7325.

Seventh Generation, 49 Hercules Drive, Colchester, VT 05446-1672; 800-456-1177.

Vermont Country Store, Box 3000, Manchester Center, VT 05255; 802-362-2400.

Index

For A Livable Planet

About Mothers & Others

Mothers & Others for a Livable Planet, conceived in 1989 by parents concerned about the impact of the environment's deterioration on the health and well-being of children, is a national nonprofit education organization working to promote consumer choices that are safe and ecologically sustainable for current and future generations. By providing strategies that can reduce individual and community consumption of natural resources, and by mobilizing consumers to seek sustainable choices in the marketplace, we aim to effect lasting protection of public health and the environment.

For only $25, members receive a one-year subscription to *The Green Guide*, the nation's premier green consumer newsletter; legislative and program updates; free consumer information; and discounts on M&O publications and products.

....

Sign me up for membership in Mothers & Others!

– putting information in your hands and power in your choices –

NAME _____

ADDRESS _____

CITY _____ **STATE** _____ **ZIP** _____

_____ $25 (basic)   _____ $50 (family)

_____ $100 (minimum for businesses)   Other $ _____

Mothers & Others • 40 West 20th Street, 9th Floor • New York, NY 10011
212-242-0010 • 1-888-ECO-INFO

tape here

tape here

To Join:

We're asking you to use this self-mailing form in order that we might spare trees and your membership dollars.

1. Fill out the renewal form on the reverse side
2. Fold where indicated
3. Enclose your check
4. Tape it shut
5. Mail it back to us!

fold

stamp

MOTHERS & OTHERS
40 W 20 ST, FL 9
NEW YORK NY 10011-4211